The Hands-on Guide to
Diabetes Care in Hospital

# The Hands-on Guide to Diabetes Care in Hospital

**David Levy**
Consultant Physician, Gillian Hanson Centre
Barts Health, Whipps Cross University Hospital
Honorary Senior Lecturer
Queen Mary University of London
London, UK

**WILEY** Blackwell

# Contents

# Preface

The much-delayed onset of concern about diabetes in hospital patients in the UK dates to 2009–10, when the now disbanded National Patient Safety Agency perceptively alerted us to poor practice, especially in insulin treatment, that had led to episodes of significant patient harm. Various insulin training modules appeared shortly after to increase awareness of hospital staff to diabetes management, and I developed one for our own hospital's training schedule. In the end, though, I think Information Governance (or it may have been Slips, Trips and Falls) was thought to be a more pressing must-do topic for gloomy 'stat and mand' training than safe insulin administration, another perverse consequence of authoritarian centralisation, especially when harm resulting from insulin misadministration is, rightly, regarded as a 'never' event. As I write this preface, however, I understand the Care Quality Commission is planning to ensure that all hospitals have an insulin safety programme in place when they pay a visit.

App mania was then at its height, and together with a young programmer friend, Adam Cubitt (Existential Ltd), who was taking some time out from animating impossible objects in multidimensional space, we set out to put the module into a more jazzy format, and to extend it to cover other important aspects of diabetes care in hospital. Our App for the iPhone and iPad (*Diabetes in Practice*) was launched in April 2012 to almost complete indifference (apart from the people administering Apple's byzantine regulatory system). I can proudly declare that worldwide our 18 months of effort have been translated into 108 downloads. Angry Birds will be relieved to learn that they won't become an endangered species on account of our foray into Appland.

Given the continuing concern about the safety of diabetic patients in hospital, which the valuable NaDIA audit in the UK continues to highlight (and which also reminds us that 15–20% of all hospital inpatients have diabetes), I thought the practical aspects of diabetes management needed a wider audience. Elizabeth Walker at Wiley Blackwell enthusiastically took on the project, and a group of trainee doctors reviewed the proposal in detail. Among other insights, they told me that I used too many words (sadly my historical fate is unlikely to be that of Mozart, of whom you may remember his patron Emperor Joseph II complained in *Amadeus*: 'Too many notes').

We have also had to diverge over the question of 'protocols', a proper discussion of which would occupy a volume three times the size of the current book. The difficulty with diabetes is that no patient ever requires exactly the same treatment, especially where insulin is concerned. This statement is not intended to establish diabetes at the pinnacle of some fantasy edifice of unfathomability or complexity. Nor is it false modesty: a most eminent professor of endocrinology whose registrar post I was quite keen on acquiring told me, as they could in the 1990s, that 'you can teach monkeys to do diabetes'. But it highlights a problem of modern medicine and its teaching, which is that skills acquisition is now deemed to be mostly independent of experience: the inevitable cry goes up, then: 'give me the protocol'.

So I have, wherever possible and safe. There *are* protocolisable bits of diabetes: the set piece hyperglycaemic emergencies, for example, and these are reflected, I hope, in precise suggestions, accompanied by the panoply of guideline medicine adjuncts, flow charts, tables and diagrams, which people tell me help them. Most of these are elaborations of the welcome guidelines produced by the Joint British Diabetes Societies Inpatient Group over the past few years. While I recognise the need for a precise and fairly dogmatic approach when managing an acutely presenting sick or problematic patient, the majority of diabetes management in hospital is more subtle and less urgent, and much of the book is in more traditional format, though I hope the topics addressed are practically relevant, and no section – other than the one on infection, for which I won't apologise – is more than about 2000 words (which is still, I know, stretching contemporary attention spans, but humour me).

Another area I have insisted on retaining is preparing for discharge and diabetes in the community. The narrowness of medical education is highlighted by the still astonishingly intact barrier between primary and secondary care. Thousands of worthy and wordy documents haven't had much impact on this, but there are places where integrated diabetes is actually happening, and patients are much better off for it. However, the idea that we can discharge a patient with a lifelong condition 'into the community' with no regard for their continuing management and welfare, especially when at least 50% of hospital trainees will have a happy and fruitful career in general practice, is, to use the technical term, bonkers.

I have tried to cover most of the practical problems that trainees will encounter, and I hope this results in a book that is apparently unconventional in parts. In particular, in a world where medical education has in some senses failed our trainees, senior physicians now have, I believe, a duty to disclose some of the 'tricks of their specialty' that they acquired during their in many cases unnecessarily long training in the 1980s and 1990s. That's quite a tall order for most consultants, who understandably still wish to maintain something of Dr House's mystique and maverick. But if we are to deliver safe – and improving – care to patients under constraints of shortened and more rigid undergraduate and postgraduate medical training, senior doctors have to loosen up and be willing to share our knowledge and experience databases. This is a legacy concern of, I think, more than trivial moment. It is currently in evidence when I see chapters written in conventional textbooks by endocrinologists who I deeply respect as clinicians, but who nevertheless revert to plonky passive prose, pathophysiological niceties, usually centring on their pet research topics, and whose voice I can't discern when I read their contributions (one of the nice things said to me about the Third Edition of *Practical Diabetes Care* (2011) was that readers could hear me speaking when they read it, a source of continuing pleasure; less pleasurable was the realisation that their education seemed to have stopped at the end of the Preface, a fate I hope won't befall this volume). Because I trust nobody will read from start to finish, there is some repetition where I think points are important but vary slightly in emphasis and context according to the clinical scenario.

The book is in pocket size, an evolutionary vestige from the remote times when white coat pockets were stuffed with these volumes. However, I hope it will find a place in the cutesy and stylish bags that trainees carry with them these days. Please send me suggestions and comments; though I recently retired from full-time work in the NHS, there is that golden period of a few years when the amyloid hasn't taken hold, so there is still a possibility of a revision or second edition before I enter Dotage from the suburbs of Cranksville.

One of my pre-consultant-period mentors, one of the great clinical diabetologists, Dr Peter Watkins of King's College Hospital, reminded me during one of his last diabetes clinics before his own retirement that he remained as fascinated and puzzled by diabetes as he had when starting his career; having trodden a similar path, I can confirm that his view remains as astute 20 years on.

Lots of people helped me. Specifically, Laura Liew supported and pushed, according to circumstance and deadline, and is responsible for much of the practical detail, including many of the clinical photographs. Dr Sergei Kuzmich, a fine radiologist at Whipps Cross University Hospital, sourced some characteristic and important films, and supplied their captions together with those dinky and all-important arrows and arrowheads. Dr Francesco Papalia (Barts Heart Centre) did some detailed research for the sections on diabetes and the heart. Ching Yee Ngan, Medicines Optimisation Pharmacist at Barts Health, supplied the valuable information on antibiotic dosing and adjustments in renal impairment. My dear colleagues in the Gillian Hanson Centre for Diabetes and Endocrinology at Whipps Cross University Hospital ('merged' into Barts Health in 2012), especially Clency Payaneandee and Joni Devine, specialist podiatrists, and Bhavanee Manogaraan and Betty Barron, specialist diabetes nurses, supported, educated and humoured me; Timo Pilgram in the Healthcare Library, or Knowledge Services, or whatever its new name is in 2015, sourced documents and papers in an electronic blink of the eye, and retitled them with scurrilous good humour (sadly they have had to revert to their pristine state for the book). It is conventional to thank patients, but without them our knowledge rarely goes beyond the confines of textbook platitudes, and nearly every insight in this book that can't be referenced is attributable to their stories and deep understanding of their condition. So, ask your patients the right questions, talk to them, accept with grateful humility that many of them know a whole lot more about diabetes than you (at least before you have studied this book), and then, of course, consult the following pages.

David Levy
*London*
*August 2015*

# Abbreviations

| | |
|---|---|
| ACE-i | Angiotensin converting enzyme inhibitor |
| ACR | Albumin : creatinine ratio |
| ACS | Acute coronary syndrome |
| AKI | Acute kidney injury |
| ARB | Angiotensin receptor blocker |
| BG | Blood glucose |
| BMS | Bare metal stent |
| CABG | Coronary artery bypass graft |
| CAD | Coronary artery disease |
| CBD | Common bile duct |
| CBG | Capillary blood glucose |
| CHO | Carbohydrate |
| CKD | Chronic kidney disease |
| CRP | C-reactive protein |
| DES | Drug-eluting stent |
| DKA | Diabetic ketoacidosis |
| DSN | Diabetes specialist nurse |
| ED | Emergency department |
| ESRD | End-stage renal disease |
| GCS | Glasgow Coma Scale |
| GIK | Glucose–insulin–potassium (intravenous infusion) |
| HBO | Hyperbaric oxygen |
| HCP(s) | Health care professional(s) |
| HHS | Hyperosmolar hyperglycaemic state (previously 'HONK') |
| i.v. | Intravenous |
| KUB | Kidneys, ureter, bladder |
| MDI | Multiple-dose insulin (basal-bolus) |
| MI | Myocardial infarction |
| MRA | Magnetic resonance angiography |
| MRCP | Magnetic resonance cholangiopancreatography |
| NSTEACS | Non-ST-elevation acute coronary syndrome |
| PCI | Percutaneous coronary intervention |
| PUO | Pyrexia of unknown origin |
| RCT(s) | Randomised controlled trial(s) |
| s.c. | Subcutaneous |
| STEMI | ST-elevation myocardial infarction |
| SU | Sulfonylurea |
| USS | Ultrasound scan |
| VBG | Venous blood gases |
| VRIII | Variable Rate Intravenous Insulin Infusion ('sliding scale' (UK) or 'insulin drip' (USA)) |

# PART 1
# Basics

# 1 Classification of diabetes

**Key points**

- Diabetes is either Type 1 or Type 2. No other terms for these major categories are permitted
- The formal diagnosis is not always obvious in acutely admitted patients (either newly diagnosed or not previously fully characterised)
- Apart from patients with DKA, you will not encounter Type 1 patients very often; this makes it especially important to identify them, as their management is completely different from that of most Type 2 patients
- Among the other specific types of diabetes (of which there are many, mostly rare), two concern the acute hospital practitioner:
  - Pancreatic
  - Drug-induced

## PHENOTYPIC FEATURES OF CLASSICAL TYPE 1 AND TYPE 2 DIABETES

Increasing numbers of people with diabetes do not conform to the stereotypes (**Figure 1.1**). Autoimmune (Type 1) diabetes occurs in older adults and Type 2 diabetes in younger adults and increasingly, though still in very small numbers in the UK, in adolescents. Some mental flexibility is needed to accommodate these – but they are clinically important because of the hazards of unexpected insulin deficiency (ketosis and the need for insulin treatment). Some scenarios are shown in **Box 1.1**.

**Classical Type 1 diabetes**
- Onset in childhood, young adulthood
- Not overweight
- Weak family history
- White ethnicity
- 100% insulin treated immediately from onset and indefinitely
- Autoimmune β-cell destruction

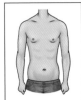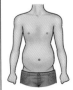

**Classical Type 2 diabetes**
- Onset in middle age
- Central obesity (mean BMI in UK 28)
- Strong family history
- Minority ethnicity (especially South Asian in UK)
- 30% insulin treated
- Non-autoimmune β-cell dysfunction + peripheral insulin resistance

**Figure 1.1** Key clinical features of classical (textbook) Type 1 and Type 2 diabetes.

*The Hands-on Guide to Diabetes Care in Hospital*, First Edition by David Levy.
© 2016 John Wiley & Sons, Ltd. Published 2016 by John Wiley & Sons, Ltd.

> **Box 1.1**   Clinical scenarios that can help in making a diagnosis
>
> - Someone on full insulin treatment alone (a regimen that covers night-time and meal times without non-insulin agents) is probably Type 1
> - Exception: some patients with very long duration Type 2 diabetes (often thin, with pancreatic 'exhaustion') take only insulin
> - Most Type 2 patients on full insulin usually take metformin as well (they may also take inject- able GLP-1 analogues and a variety of oral agents; see **Chapter 24**)
> - Someone on full insulin since childhood, adolescence, or early adulthood (up to 30–35) is Type 1. Most patients can remember accurately how long they have been taking insulin. Late- onset Type 1 diabetes can occur at any age (often in people with a strong personal or family history of associated autoimmune conditions)
> - Northern Europe (especially UK and Scandinavia), Australia and New Zealand have the highest incidence of Type 1 diabetes
> - A non-overweight white person of *any* age treated with insulin alone has Type 1 diabetes. Many people now survive without significant complications for 50 years or more (they will be in their 60s and 70s). They often need only tiny doses of insulin (e.g. <20 units/day) but are still insulin-requiring and ketosis-prone
> - Thin people are likely to have Type 1 diabetes, but there are a lot of overweight Type 1 pa- tients who have insulin-resistant features and may require high-dose insulin

There is a small proportion (around 5%) with unusual forms of diabetes (e.g. domi- nantly inherited monogenic forms, previously termed maturity-onset diabetes of the young (MODY); syndromic diabetes; pancreatic diabetes). Patients with pancreatic dia- betes are usually insulin-requiring (and ketosis-prone), but technically not Type 1, as β-cell destruction is caused by non-autoimmune processes, e.g. alcohol, calcification.

## Terminology

Table 1.1 shows the several obsolete terms for diabetes, but they still turn up depress- ingly often (as I write this, a cohort of trainees has taken to using IDDM and NIDDM, terms that were outdated about 14 years ago). 'IDDM' and 'NIDDM' roll off the tongue very easily (just like 'BM': see **Chapter 4**) but that's no reason to use them.

This is NOT nitpicking. Withdrawing insulin (omission in the clinical context) in Type 1 di- abetic patients may result in severe ketosis within 4 hours (e.g. plasma β-hydroxybutyrate around 3 mmol/L) in the absence of especially high blood glucose levels (e.g. 14–15 mmol/L).

**Table 1.1** Alternative terms for Type 1 and Type 2 diabetes

| Type 1 | Type 2 | Comments |
|---|---|---|
| Type I | Type II | Use Arabic, not Roman numerals, National Diabetes Data Group (NDDG), 2003 |
| Insulin-dependent | Non-insulin-dependent | Declared obsolete, 2003 (NDDG) |
| IDDM | NIDDM | Declared obsolete, 2003 (NDDG). It's hazardous to use IDDM to describe any insulin-taking patient, most of whom are Type 2 |
| Juvenile-onset | Adult onset, maturity-onset | Very obsolete, but more descriptive and precise than other terms |
| Ketosis-prone | Non-ketosis-prone | 'Ketosis-prone diabetes' is coming back into use to describe patients who at onset are insulin-deficient; this group includes 'Flatbush' diabetes (Type 2), and fulminant diabetes (Type 1B). The full new classification (Aβ) requires measurements of markers of islet-cell autoimmunity (A) and β-cell function (β), neither of which are routinely available |
| | 'Sugar diabetes', 'A touch of diabetes', 'Mild diabetes' | • 'Sugar diabetes' is rarely used except by people and physicians of a certain age.<br>• 'A touch of diabetes' is an elegant phrase, but has no quantitative basis.<br>• 'Mild diabetes' was a clinically acceptable term for well-controlled Type 2 diabetes before Type 1 and Type 2 were distinguished. Generally deplored now, but some forms of Type 2 diabetes run a benign course with excellent long-term control on minimal or no medication |
| | Diet-controlled diabetes | A precise term – when it's true. 'Diet-treated diabetes' is a better starting point, pending assessment of CBGs and HbA$_{1c}$. Most Type 2 patients require medication |

# 2 Targets for glycaemic control in hospital

**Key points**

The target for blood glucose levels in all adult patients in hospital is

**7–10 mmol/L**

**This target applies to:**

- All general medical and surgical patients, including those on artificial nutrition or steroids (see **Chapters 28 and 29**)
- Post-MI patients
- Post-stroke patients
- Patients on ICU/HDU
- Persistent hyperglycaemia (blood glucose >12–15 mmol/L) may increase infection risk, especially postoperative, but hypoglycaemia (blood glucose <4.0 mmol/L) is probably more hazardous (strong hint of increased risk of mortality in the year after discharge).
- These are consensus values, as there is little randomised controlled trial (RCT) evidence for these targets. However, there are high-quality studies in adults (NICE-SUGAR, 2009) and children (Macrae et al. 2014) in ICU that show clearly there is no benefit in tight glucose control (e.g. BG 4–7 mmol/L) compared with less tight control (e.g. <10–12 mmol/L).

## MYOCARDIAL INFARCTION (Chapters 13 and 14)

**There are two considerations:**

**1. Target blood glucose levels**: desirable blood glucose levels for MI patients are not known. The famous DIGAMI study (Malmberg et al. 1997) initiated insulin treatment at BG >11.1 mmol/L, that is at a level diagnostic of diabetes

**2. Treatment**: is insulin of benefit compared with any other treatments? (Theoretically insulin increases myocardial metabolic efficiency, converting fatty acid to glucose metabolism.) Inpatient intravenous insulin in DIGAMI was followed by 3 months of intensive subcutaneous insulin, but with limited benefits – fatal infarction fell by 11%, but reinfarction rates did not change

- The indications for i.v. insulin in MI patients are the same as for other medical patients (critical illness, nil by mouth)
- Do not discontinue metformin unless there are contraindications (**Chapter 24**)
- All other glucose-lowering agents can be used

---

*The Hands-on Guide to Diabetes Care in Hospital*, First Edition by David Levy.
© 2016 John Wiley & Sons, Ltd. Published 2016 by John Wiley & Sons, Ltd.

# STROKE

Blood glucose targets have not been established. Manage elevated BG levels in the same way as MI patients. Insulin is of no value and may cause hypoglycaemia, a concern in patients who may have fluctuating and impaired awareness.

# ICU/HDU

From 2000–2008, tight glycaemic control was widely advocated after a series of studies in Belgium found some prognostic benefit in surgical patients (BG levels 4–6 compared with 10–11 mmol/L). In general ICU patients, the same level of tight control increased mortality, compared with targeting <10 mmol/L, and there was a high rate of moderate and severe hypoglycaemia (NICE-SUGAR). A target BG 7–10 mmol/L is generally now advised.

# SURGICAL PATIENTS (Chapter 27)

There are no robust randomized controlled trials (RCTs), but countless retrospective studies that associate increased BG levels with increased risk of postoperative infection. There are no studies comparing insulin with other agents.

## References

Macrae D, Grieve R, Allen E, et al.; CHiP Investigators. A randomized trial of hyperglycaemic control in pediatric intensive care. *N Engl J Med.* 2014;370:107–18. PMID: 24401049.

Malmberg K; DIGAMI (Diabetes Mellitus, Insulin Glucose Infusion in Acute Myocardial Infarction) Study Group. Prospective randomised study of intensive insulin treatment on long term survival after acute myocardial infarction in patients with diabetes mellitus. *BMJ.* 1997;314:1512–15. PMID: 9169397.

NICE-SUGAR Study Investigators; Finfer S, Chittock DR, Su SY, et al. Intensive versus conventional glucose control in critically ill patients. *N Engl J Med.* 2009;360:1283–97. PMID: 19318384.

# 3 Diagnosis of diabetes in hospitalised patients

| Diagnostic criteria | |
| --- | --- |
| Random glucose | >11.1 mmol/L |
| Fasting glucose | ≥7.0 mmol/L |
| HbA$_{1c}$ | ≥6.5% (48 mmol/mol) |

Blood glucose measurements should ideally be laboratory (venous plasma), but in acute hospital practice capillary blood glucose (CBG) measurements are acceptable. It would be wise to confirm measurements that are near threshold values (7 or 11 mmol/L) with laboratory measurements. When making a diagnosis always take a specimen for HbA$_{1c}$, even though you may not get the result back during a short admission; it is widely accepted as a diagnostic test, and given the frequency of undiagnosed diabetes in hospitalised patients, it should be requested more often. A formal diagnosis is of benefit both to the patient and their primary care team (**Figure 3.1**).

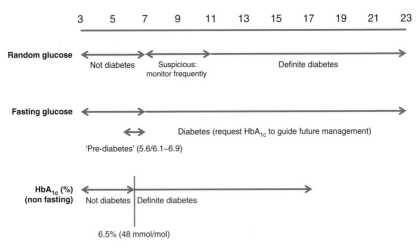

**Figure 3.1** Criteria for diagnosing diabetes in hospitalised patients using random and fasting glucose levels, and HbA$_{1c}$.

*The Hands-on Guide to Diabetes Care in Hospital,* First Edition by David Levy.
© 2016 John Wiley & Sons, Ltd. Published 2016 by John Wiley & Sons, Ltd.

## STRESS HYPERGLYCAEMIA

Blood glucose levels in hospital that are diagnostic of diabetes, on a background of normal glucose levels (i.e. non-diabetic $HbA_{1c}$ – <6.5%, 48 mmol/mol). It is a valuable diagnosis for the patient as it will help management in the medium term once out of hospital. Though interesting, it is not often looked for, but does not detract from the importance of treating hyperglycaemia during the current admission.

# 4 Nomenclature

- Capillary blood glucose (CBG)
- 'Sliding scale' insulin/insulin drip/ Variable Rate Intravenous Insulin Infusion (VRIII)
- HbA$_{1c}$ (glycated haemoglobin)

## CAPILLARY BLOOD GLUCOSE

In the UK, the term 'BM' is frequently used as a substitute for the true description of a blood glucose measurement of capillary blood obtained by finger prick – capillary blood glucose (CBG). (Boehringer–Mannheim were the manufacturers of a pioneering but long-obsolete colour-coded blood glucose test strip.) In the UK 'BM' has installed itself with depressing grimness and no sign of disappearing from use, even by senior clinicians who should know better. It is akin in illogicality to referring to a peak flow rate as an 'MW' (Mini-Wright, a widely used meter in the UK) rather than L/min. It is also medico-legally ambiguous. Resolve to expunge this silly abbreviation from your jargon outbox, and wag your finger at consultants who indulge in the same sloppiness. CBG is fully acceptable.

## VRIII (VARIABLE RATE INTRAVENOUS INSULIN INFUSION, 'SLIDING SCALE' IN THE UK)

'Sliding scale' is a slithery term, and the Joint British Diabetes Societies have wisely decided to abandon it and replace it with the more accurate Variable Rate Intravenous Insulin Infusion (VRIII). The Americans use 'sliding scale' to describe a traditional but ineffective method of giving *subcutaneous* soluble insulin (without basal insulin) in response to postprandial blood glucose measurements in hospitalised patients. The North American term for VRIII, 'insulin drip', is better than 'sliding scale'. See **Chapter 17** for further discussion of indications for VRIII.

## HbA$_{1c}$ (GLYCATED HAEMOGLOBIN)

Request an HbA$_{1c}$ measurement on every diabetic person who comes into the hospital, as well as people just about to start glucocorticoid treatment and enteral feeding (both of which can precipitate severe hyperglycaemia even in people not known to have diabetes; **Chapters 28** and **29**). If you're concerned about cost, substitute a single HbA$_{1c}$ measurement for one day's ritual request for CRP or LFTs. Most laboratories will process HbA$_{1c}$ requests only two or three times a week, so you may not get the result back during a short admission. This shouldn't be a reason not to request it (autoantibodies

*The Hands-on Guide to Diabetes Care in Hospital,* First Edition by David Levy.
© 2016 John Wiley & Sons, Ltd. Published 2016 by John Wiley & Sons, Ltd.

are requested almost as frequently as HbA$_{1c}$ with much less chance of the results being back during an admission).

Glycation is the process of mostly irreversible nonenzymatic attachment of a glucose molecule to the N-terminal of the β-chain of the haemoglobin molecule that occurs over the lifespan of the red cell, and therefore represents glycaemic control over a period of 6–10 weeks before the test. The ratio of glycated haemoglobin to total haemoglobin gave rise to the familiar percentage measurement (DCCT measurement, usual range 6–12%) in universal use since the late 70s. Latterly a massive bureaucratic upheaval in the upper echelons of clinical biochemistry proposed a change to using only the IFCC measurement, which would ultimately be traceable to an absolute standard, hence the new ratio expressed in molar concentrations (usual range 42–108 mmol/mol). There is no easy conversion between the two measures, other than to remember that 8% = 64 mmol//L and that 1% = 11 mmol/mol. Much of the world has regarded the new measurement as too troublesome to implement with only marginal benefits for patients, and most countries are still reporting in both units. The majority of clinicians and patients have little or no accurate feel for the new units more than 3 years after its implementation in the UK, though in acute medical practice the nuances of small changes are of less importance. A conversion table, with associated estimated average glucose (eAG) levels, is shown in **Table 4.1**.

Table 4.1   HbA$_{1c}$ conversion, together with approximate corresponding estimated average glucose measurements (eAG) and 95% confidence intervals. Note that the target range for inpatient glucose levels (7–10 mmol/L) corresponds to an HbA$_{1c}$ ~7%, which is lower than the average outpatient population measurement (~8%). Strict normoglycaemia (non-diabetic-range glucose measurements) corresponds to HbA$_{1c}$ ~5% (from Nathan et al., 2008).

| HbA$_{1c}$ | | eAG | |
|---|---|---|---|
| DCCT (%) | IFCC (mmol/mol) | (mmol/L) | (mg/dL) |
| 6 | 42 | 7.0   (5.5–8.5) | 126   (100–152) |
| 7 | 53 | 8.6   (6.8–10.3) | 154   (123–185) |
| 8 | 64 | 10.2   (8.1–12.1) | 183   (147–217) |
| 9 | 75 | 11.8   (9.4–13.9) | 212   (170–249) |
| 10 | 86 | 13.4   (10.7–15.7) | 240   (193–282) |
| 11 | 97 | 14.9   (12.0–17.5) | 269   (217–314) |
| 12 | 108 | 16.5   (13.3–19.3) | 298   (240–347) |
| 13 | 119 | 18.1   (15–21) | 326   (260–380) |
| 14 | 130 | 19.7   (16–23) | 355   (290–410) |
| 15 | 140 | 21.3   (17–25) | 384   (310–440) |

## Low HbA$_{1c}$ in older people, 65 years or over, with Type 2 diabetes

Although inpatients often have very poor glucose levels as a cause or a result of their admission, recall that many community patients, most of them treated with insulin or sulphonylureas, have low HbA$_{1c}$ levels (<7.0%, 53 mmol/mol; Lipska et al., 2015). This proportion, around 60%, at least in the USA, has not changed over more than 10 years, is approximately the same for people in good general health and those with multiple co-morbidities alike, and puts many older people, especially in the latter group, at risk of hypoglycaemia. Recognise the potential adverse consequences of such low levels, and if you encounter it, reduce culprit medications, especially sulphonylureas, and explicitly mention it in discharge summaries.

### 'Burnt-out' diabetes in advanced kidney disease

A graphic but imprecise term, describing near-normal blood glucose levels in patients with CKD stages 4 and 5. Very common, but not widely recognised: around 65% of dialysis patients have $HbA_{1c}$ <7.0% (53 mmol/mol), and 35% <6.0% (42 mmol/mol). These levels confer no prognostic benefit: diabetic maculopathy and peripheral and autonomic neuropathy do not improve with ultra-tight glycaemic control at this stage of diabetes. Many patients with longstanding diabetes resulting in ESRD have associated advanced autonomic neuropathy, hypoglycaemia unawareness and severe CHD. Hypoglycaemia in this group is common, severe and may be associated with arrhythmic death. The causes are multiple (**Box 4.1**) but in practice, ensure CBG levels are consistently no lower than 7–10 mmol/L, by excluding all agents contraindicated in renal failure (see **Chapter 24**), and reducing insulin doses. Because the low blood glucose levels are not due just to medication, even when all hypoglycaemic drugs are discontinued, patients may still have nearly non-diabetic blood glucose levels. Don't make the problem worse by a misplaced insistence on 'good' glycaemic control with multiple medications. Despite their many co-morbidities (visual impairment, immobility, amputations and heart failure) try to make special efforts to involve them with hospital or community diabetes specialist nurses in ensuring follow-up so that diabetes medication can be minimised. In addition, don't underestimate the psychological benefit of withdrawing some medication from these patients who may be taking a massive number of drugs.

---

**Box 4.1**   Factors contributing to 'burnt-out' diabetes

- Prescribed medications
- Decreased renal insulin degradation and clearance
- Declining renal gluconeogenesis
- Decreased food intake and loss of lean body mass and fat (patients can gradually lose substantial amounts of weight, though they are often still overweight)

---

## References

Lipska KJ, Ross JS, Miao Y, Shah ND, Lee SJ, Steinman MA. Potential overtreatment of diabetes mellitus in older adults with tight glycemic control. *JAMA Intern Med.* 2015;75:356–62. PMID: 25581565.

Nathan DM, Kuenen J, Borg R, Zheng H, Schoenfeld D, Heine RJ; A1c-Derived Average Glucose Study Group. Translating the A1C assay into estimated average glucose values. *Diabetes Care.* 2008;31:1473–8. PMID: 18540046.

**Web conversion between DCCT and IFCC $HbA_{1c}$ values**
   www.diabetes.co.uk/hba1c-units-converter.html (accessed on 26 August 2015)

# 5 Outline of physiology

## INSULIN ACTIONS

Insulin is the major endogenous anabolic hormone, with primary effects on glucose lowering and converting glucose to the storage forms of glycogen and fat in insulin-sensitive tissues. Biochemical actions are shown in **Figure 5.1**; **Table 5.1** shows the effects on processes. Insulin deficiency (as in newly presenting Type 1 diabetes or diabetic ketoacidosis (DKA)) causes carbohydrate, fat and protein catabolism.

**Table 5.1** Insulin actions on metabolism

|  | Insulin | | |
|---|---|---|---|
|  | Activates | Inhibits | Effect of insulin deficiency |
| **Glucose** | Glucose uptake in muscle, adipose tissue and liver | Gluconeogenesis | Hyperglycaemia |
| **Glycogen** | Glycogen synthesis | Glycogenolysis | Hyperglycaemia |
| **Lipids** | Fatty acid uptake and triglyceride synthesis | Lipolysis | Hypertriglyceridaemia → ↑ Non-esterified fatty acids (NEFA) → ketosis |
| **Protein** | Protein synthesis | Proteolysis | Muscle wasting prominent in chronic insulin deficiency |
| **Ionic effects** | Uptake of ions (especially $K^+$ and $PO_4$) |  | Hyperkalaemia |

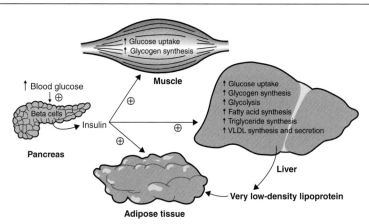

**Figure 5.1** The major actions of insulin in insulin-sensitive tissues (adipose, liver and muscle) serving to reduce blood glucose levels. *Source*: Coffee 1998. Reproduced with permission of Wiley.

*The Hands-on Guide to Diabetes Care in Hospital,* First Edition by David Levy.
© 2016 John Wiley & Sons, Ltd. Published 2016 by John Wiley & Sons, Ltd.

## DIABETIC KETOACIDOSIS (Chapter 9)

Insulin deficiency results in increased non-esterified free fatty acids, which are then metabolised in hepatic mitochondria by β-oxidation to ketone bodies (Figure 5.2).

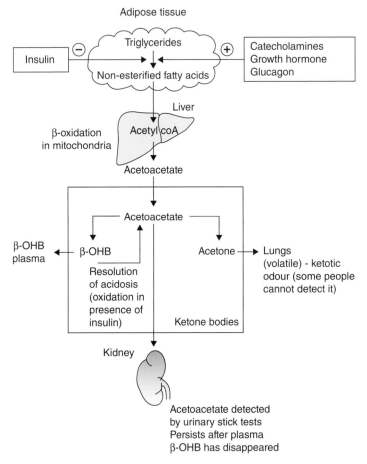

**Figure 5.2** Ketone body metabolism in diabetic ketoacidosis. Acetoacetate persists in the urine (and is detected by routine stick testing) long after DKA resolves as monitored by the predominant acid-forming ketone body, β-hydroxybutyrate. Measuring capillary blood ketones often allows i.v. insulin infusions to be discontinued earlier and more safely without the risk of 'rebound' ketosis. *Source:* Levy 2011. Reproduced with permission of Wiley. β-OHB: β-hydroxybutyrate.

# INSULIN RESISTANCE

Insulin resistance = resistance to insulin-mediated glucose uptake in insulin sensitive tissues (liver, muscle and fat).

How insulin resistance contributes to Type 2 diabetes (and it plays a part in some patients with Type 1 diabetes as well) has been discussed for decades. The clinical associations of chronic insulin resistance, for example, polycystic ovarian syndrome and non-alcoholic fatty liver disease, do not concern the acute physician, but it has several important consequences for the management of unwell inpatients:

**1.** Increased insulin requirements in insulin-treated patients
**2.** The need for insulin treatment in ill and postoperative patients, especially with infections
**3.** Acute insulin resistance caused by glucocorticoids

## RENAL DISEASE

Injected insulin is not degraded by first-pass metabolism in the liver, and although it is freely filtered by the kidney it is nearly all reabsorbed and metabolised by renal tissue, so that <1% of an injected dose is excreted. Diabetic nephropathy is usually associated with insulin resistance and high insulin requirements. However, below an eGFR of 20 mL/min, insulin clearance decreases, its half-life increases, insulin requirements fall and there is a risk of hypoglycaemia. Many patients have additional risk factors for hypoglycaemia unawareness, for example long duration of diabetes, autonomic neuropathy.

## HYPEROSMOLAR HYPERGLYCAEMIC STATE

The pathophysiology of the hyperosmolar hyperglycaemic state (HHS) is not fully understood, and is likely to differ between patients, as insulin resistance and insulin deficiency in different measures contribute to Type 2 diabetes.

The idea of 'partial insulin deficiency' explains why ketosis is usually absent in HHS patients. Suppression of lipolysis requires lower insulin concentrations than glucose uptake into tissues. Slowly progressing hyperglycaemia without the acute disturbances caused by ketosis accounts for the longer prodromal period of HHS compared with DKA.

## HYPOGLYCAEMIA (Chapters 11 and 26)

Counter-regulation in the non-diabetic person (reduced endogenous insulin secretion, increased glucagon) occurs when BG levels fall below ~3.8 mmol/L (Figure 5.3). With further reductions the sequence of further endocrine counter-regulatory activation is stereotyped, but clinical symptoms may be less so, and the character of symptoms changes significantly with increasing duration of diabetes, especially in Type 1. While many patients will be unaware of symptoms at 4 mmol/L, it is the sound basis for the useful educational mnemonic 'four's the floor', though the slogan loses some of its punch when expressed in traditional units (4 mmol/L = 72 mg/dL). Cognitive function is invariably impaired at BG <3.0 mmol/L.

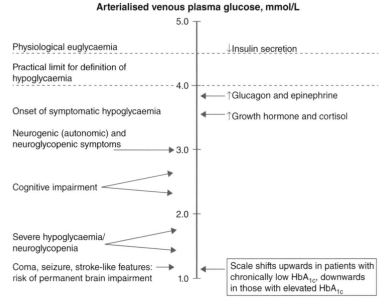

**Figure 5.3**  Physiological, clinical and counter-regulatory responses to insulin-induced hypoglycaemia. *Source*: Levy 2011. Reproduced with permission of Wiley.

## Further reading

Coffee CJ. *Metabolism*. Fence Creek Publishing, 1998.
Frayn, KN. *Metabolic Regulation: A Human Perspective*, 3rd edn. Wiley-Blackwell, 2010.
Levy D. *Practical Diabetes Care*, 3rd edn. Wiley-Blackwell, 2011.

# 6 Diabetes specialist nurses: roles and responsibilities

Get to know your hospital diabetes specialist nurses (DSNs) and what they expect of you (and your team); they are the key professionals responsible for managing most inpatient diabetes, and you can learn a lot from them about the practical management of diabetes problems. They are also masters of up-to-date technology, from insulin identification cards to subcutaneous insulin pumps. Their numbers, seniority, affiliations and responsibilities vary widely between hospitals. Some are prescribers and increasingly in the UK dedicated inpatient diabetes nurses (without outpatient responsibilities) are part of an inpatient diabetes team (DSN, endocrine registrar and consultant). In many (but not all) hospitals, you, and not DSNs, will be expected to initially see ED and emergency admission unit patients with acutely presenting problems. DSNs will usually liaise with community diabetes and general nursing services when a patient is discharged (e.g. patients newly started on insulin who need district nurses to give insulin).

Because up to 20% of inpatients have diabetes (that means upwards of 100 patients at any time in many hospitals) and the majority were not admitted with a primary diabetes problem, there are too many patients for a usual small team of DSNs to regularly review all of them. In many hospitals, therefore, you will be expected to:

- Initiate non-insulin treatments
- Modify non-insulin treatments and insulin, according to blood glucose monitoring results
- Identify recurrent hypoglycaemia and reduce medication and insulin accordingly
- Refer patients appropriately if they have diabetes-related problems (e.g. renal, foot, acute eye problems)
- Liaise with them if patients have consistent hyperglycaemia or recurrent hypoglycaemia that is not responding to rational treatment changes
- Take their advice if it is asked for (they are senior colleagues and may not appreciate ritual referrals just because a patient has diabetes, and your hospital will not appreciate your keeping well-controlled patients in hospital in order to be 'reviewed' by them)
- Discuss with them (much better in person) if you have any questions or problems managing diabetes in hospital patients. In practice, these will be patients whose insulin regimens are evidently not appropriate (medically or difficulty in self-management)

There is a small number of nurse consultants in diabetes, who often have a more managerial than clinical role. Again, some are based in hospital, others in the community.

*The Hands-on Guide to Diabetes Care in Hospital,* First Edition by David Levy.
© 2016 John Wiley & Sons, Ltd. Published 2016 by John Wiley & Sons, Ltd.

# PART 2
# Acute diabetes problems

# 7 History taking in patients with diabetes

**Top tip**

Diabetes diagnosis, duration, complications and accurate current treatment are all you need: focus on these. Look up any recent biochemistry and HbA$_{1c}$ on the hospital system.

**Key points**

- Don't use obsolete terms for diabetes diagnoses (see **Chapter 1**). At best they can mislead, at worst they present hazard. If you don't know the type of diabetes, describe it, for example, 'diabetes, onset age 35, insulin treated since diagnosis'. The formal diagnosis can be reviewed later if necessary
- Focus on treatment. If you are seeing a patient initially with their carer, you're much more likely to get the treatment correct – they may recall more accurately than the patient, be able to get a prescription record, or contact someone immediately who *will* know the patient's treatment
- Once the patient is out of the emergency department, you are increasingly unlikely to get their diabetes treatment correct
- A few minutes spent focusing on diabetes-specific history is much more important than filling in all the boxes of systems enquiry
- Look up the hospital pathology database for a recent HbA$_{1c}$ and renal function results (very likely requested by the patient's GP)

Eliciting a good diabetes history, like any medical history, should take no more than a few minutes, but focus on the things that really matter to the patient and their safety.

## TYPE OF DIABETES/DIAGNOSIS (Chapter 1)

### Critical:

- Don't use 'IDDM' or 'NIDDM'
- Don't write 'Type 1 diabetes' just because someone is insulin treated; most insulin-treated patients have Type 2 diabetes; conversely, don't write 'Insulin-treated Type 2 diabetes' just because the patient is older; there is, happily, now a large number of Type 1 patients in their 70s and 80s
- If this *is* Type 1 diabetes, ensure the patient has not missed and will not miss *any* insulin doses (ask, and if there is uncertainty get urinary and/or ketone measurements: ketosis = insulin deficiency)

---

*The Hands-on Guide to Diabetes Care in Hospital,* First Edition by David Levy.
© 2016 John Wiley & Sons, Ltd. Published 2016 by John Wiley & Sons, Ltd.

## DURATION OF DIABETES

The 'pre-clinical' duration of Type 2 diabetes is 7–10 years – Type 2 diabetes therefore often presents with advanced diabetes complications. You can correctly state either 'Type 2 diabetes, diagnosed 1995' or 'Known duration of Type 2 diabetes 17 years'.

Type 1 diabetes nearly always has an acute clinical onset: the younger the age of diagnosis the more acute the onset. The autoimmune process becomes less intense with age, so Type 1 patients in their 30s and older with Latent Autoimmune Diabetes of Adult onset (LADA) may be controlled for a short time on tablets (the definition allows 6 months; see **Chapter 8**). Multiple factors conspire to make diabetes with onset in young adults a diagnostic and therapeutic challenge (**Figure 7.1**).

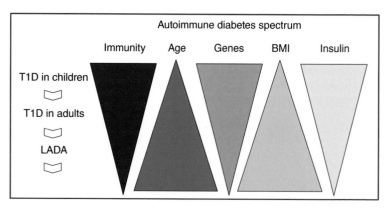

**Figure 7.1** The spectrum of autoimmune diabetes. Five known variable domains interact to generate the broadening presentation of autoimmune diabetes in younger and middle-aged people. *Source:* Reproduced with permission of Professor David Leslie, St. Bartholomew's Hospital.

### 'Honeymoon' period (remission)

A period of variable duration (usually 9–12 months) after the clinical onset of Type 1 diabetes during which insulin requirements are low or very low (~0.3–0.5 U/kg/day, sometimes as low as 0.1 U/kg/day). This is a spontaneous partial remission, the pathophysiology of which is not understood. Despite the very low doses of insulin, patients in this period after diagnosis should still be regarded as insulin-deficient and ketosis-prone; do not discontinue insulin treatment.

### Long-term Type 1 diabetes

Long-term survivors of Type 1 diabetes (>50 years duration) are as a group extremely insulin-sensitive, and have an average daily insulin requirement similar to people in honeymoon, that is around 0.5 U/kg/day. In a thin individual, this may amount to no more than about 4 units of insulin with meals, and 10 units of basal insulin. They are, nevertheless, fully insulin-requiring and ketosis-prone.

Duration of diabetes is associated with increasing risks of both micro- and macro -vascular complications. Type 1 patients rarely have microvascular complications within less than about 10 years of diagnosis, but Type 2 patients are frequently diagnosed at the same time as an acute admission with a vascular complication, especially ACS and stroke. Any patient with known diabetes duration >10 years needs careful consideration of complications.

## TREATMENT (Chapter 24)

### Oral hypoglycaemics (tablets)

Not usually a problem to identify, and none are critical in the early stages of admission. In sick Type 2 patients, try to establish whether they are currently taking metformin (always large white tablets) and in what dose because of the outside possibility of lactic acidosis.

### GLP-1 analogues

Non-insulin injectable agents, usually taken once or twice daily, sometimes weekly – always with disposable pens. Some patients think of these agents as insulin – the pen devices for GLP-1 analogues and insulin look similar.

### Insulin

Patients should carry insulin-identification cards (**Figure 7.2**) but usually don't (mostly because we do not consistently give them out or change them when insulin preparations

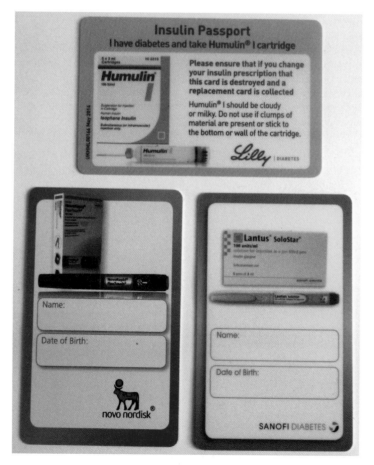

**Figure 7.2** Insulin identification cards. Plastic, credit card sized. Patients would probably carry them if we bothered to give them out (and to change them when their insulin preparations are altered).

are altered). All the major insulin companies supply them to hospitals, usually via diabetes specialist nurses. Overseas patients may take insulin preparations not available in the UK (see **Chapter 20**). Ask to see any home blood glucose monitoring records (1 mmol glucose $\cong$ 20 mg). Written diaries are usually more helpful in spotting diurnal patterns of glycaemic control, especially hypoglycaemia, than the simple chronological sequence of results stored by most blood glucose meters.

Establishing the patient's current insulin preparations and doses is critically important, but doing so can occasionally be frustrating and time-consuming. A key long-term aim of insulin treatment is patient autonomy, and many patients – including nearly all Type 1 patients – will adjust insulin dosing day-to-day and dose-to-dose according to CBG levels, activity, carbohydrate intake and intercurrent illness and stress. **There may therefore be no written record of the patient's current insulin doses – anywhere**. If there is a critical illness i.v. insulin will be needed; if there isn't, and you have no way of accurately establishing insulin doses in time for the next insulin dose, you may need to consider improvising an emergency insulin regimen (**Chapter 23**).

If the patient has any doubts about the details of their insulin treatment, ask accompanying people – carers, relatives, friends, children in the case of non-English speaking patients, and with permission look at all containers of medication (individual insulin pens tend to gravitate towards the bottom of carrier bags). You may only have one opportunity to do this before the patient is moved from the emergency department to a ward where they may need their first dose soon. Do not leave your ward-based colleague to sort out the problem. **Box 7.1** outlines some key questions that will help identify broad types of insulin, and **Figure 7.3** is a simple flow chart to help identify specific types of insulin.

---

**Box 7.1**  Key questions to help identify insulin regimens (see **Chapters 20** and **21**)

- Do you take diabetes tablets (ask specifically about metformin)?
- How many times a day do you take insulin?
  - If once a day, then likely Type 2 diabetes, taking isophane (cloudy) or long-acting analogue (clear) – usually at bedtime
  - If twice a day then probably a mixture (cloudy) taken before breakfast and evening meal; nearly always Type 2, but a few Type 1 patients use twice-daily mixtures
  - If three times a day, then possibly a mixture (cloudy) before the three meals (usually Type 2)
  - If four times a day, then if you don't know otherwise, assume the patient has Type 1 diabetes (regardless of age, ethnicity or BMI) – even though basal-bolus insulin is used in Type 2 diabetes
- Have you taken or been given your insulin doses today?
- When was the last time you had your insulin?
- Is it cloudy insulin (isophane or biphasic insulin)?

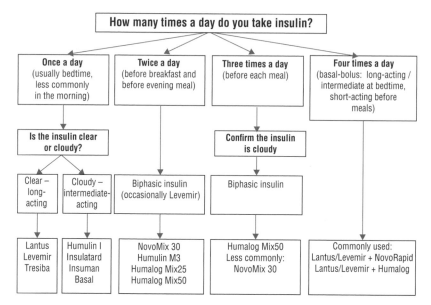

**Figure 7.3** Identifying insulin preparations based on the frequency of injections. If the patient is taking non-insulin diabetes drugs, then they very likely have Type 2 diabetes.

## COMPLICATIONS

### Retinopathy

Is the patient under the supervision of the hospital eye clinic? If so, there is either significant retinopathy – proliferative or maculopathy – requiring current treatment, or there is high-risk retinopathy, for example, preproliferative? Although the retinopathy itself will not require treatment during a non-diabetes illness, retinopathy is a reasonably reliable predictor of renal disease and clusters with many of the other micro- and macrovascular complications.

### Nephropathy

Dialysis? Peritoneal or haemo-?

Does the patient come to the renal clinic? It may be a low-clearance (pre-dialysis) clinic or a combined renal-diabetic clinic, usually for patients with CKD stage 4 or 5.

### Foot complications

Patients with active foot problems often have repeated admissions. Is the patient under active follow-up with the specialist podiatry service?

### Macrovascular disease

Type 2 patients often have complex and advanced coronary heart disease: stents, bypass. Angina symptoms are often muted or unusual (shortness of breath, non-specific chest symptoms rather than classical exertional pain; **Chapter 12**).

# 8 Assessment and initial management of patients presenting with high blood glucose levels to an emergency department

**Key points**

- It is simple, quick and good practice to exclude an imminent hyperglycaemic emergency in all patients attending ED with high blood glucose levels (usually >15–20 mmol/L)
- Most patients will as a minimum require adjustment of their diabetes medication; some will need an insulin start – perhaps soon
- If the ultimate assessment is of poorly controlled diabetes, give patients a plan in outline about next steps. Refer clearly and precisely with your clinical assessment

Many patients present to their local ED concerned about high blood glucose levels. The usual scenarios are:

- Imminent or established hyperglycaemic emergency
- Newly diagnosed patients, usually Type 2 recently started on treatment, who have been told that there is an (arbitrary) 'high' blood glucose level, above which there is cause for concern
- Newly diagnosed Type 2 patients referred by their primary care team are sometimes found to have positive urinary ketones (capillary ketone measurements are not available in primary care centres, though some Type 1 patients use reliable devices for home testing)

Your tasks – not always easy – are to:

- Discharge patients who have uncomplicated hyperglycaemia
- Rapidly assess, start treatment and arrange to admit to an appropriate area of the hospital patients with imminent or actual hyperglycaemic emergencies
- Consider factors such as emerging infection that might complicate discharge

**Figure 8.1** is a scheme for rapid assessment of patients with hyperglycaemia.

**Always admit:**
- Confirmed DKA (pH <7.3, $HCO_3$ <17, ketosis)
- Confirmed HHS (osmolarity >320 mOsmol/kg)
- Mixed HHS/DKA with complex or puzzling biochemistry (e.g. large anion gap)
- Patients with impaired consciousness (need time to evaluate whether metabolic state, other medical problem, or both is contributing)

*The Hands-on Guide to Diabetes Care in Hospital,* First Edition by David Levy.
© 2016 John Wiley & Sons, Ltd. Published 2016 by John Wiley & Sons, Ltd.

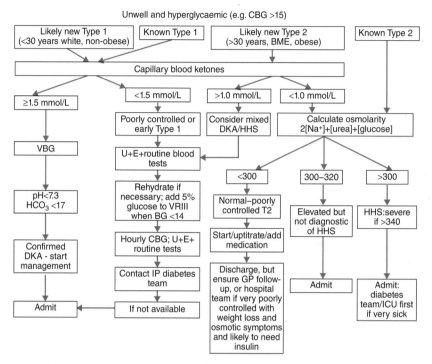

**Figure 8.1** Assessing patients who arrive at the ED with high blood glucose levels – usually >15 mmol/L. Patients with presenting glucose levels >25 are likely to need admission, possibly brief, whatever the scenario. Discharge patients only if there is adequate social support and a continuity plan. (BME = black and minority ethnic; VBG = venous blood gas)

- Insulin-treated patients who would not be able to self-administer if discharged
- Dialysis patients (high risk of underlying infection) – unless seen promptly by renal senior

## TYPE 1 DIABETES INTERCEPTED EARLY IN ITS COURSE

Although new-onset Type 1 diabetes is uncommon (outnumbered by Type 2 diabetes 20-fold), think about it in non-obese white people under 40, especially if there is no family history – though people of any ethnic group can be affected. They may not have significant ketonuria in the early stages, particularly those with later-onset autoimmune diabetes (patients in their 30s, 40s or beyond); increasing numbers can be managed on non-insulin agents while their β-cell function, presumably, is adequate, sometimes over several years. You may therefore see Type 1 diabetes that has gradually decompensated in the months before presentation. So long as there is no acute problem, they don't require admission, but you could be doing the patient a great favour by at least raising the possibility of Type 1 diabetes (many patients diagnosed over 30 are automatically labelled as Type 2). The formal diagnosis of Latent Autoimmune Diabetes of Adult onset (LADA) requires:

- Onset of non-insulin requiring diabetes over the age of 30
- Presence of islet-associated anti-GAD antibodies
- >6 months from diagnosis to requiring insulin

but this triad is of limited assistance to the acute physician, and even the first criterion is arbitrary.

### Ethnicity

Eastern European people (Baltic states [Latvia, Estonia, Lithuania], Poland, Romania, Bulgaria, Czech Republic, Hungary).

Although the risk of Type 1 diabetes in these countries is lower than in the UK, they are a young group in the UK, and they are frequently seen in urban emergency departments.

There is a high rate of associated autoimmune conditions, especially thyroid. In the past few years we have seen two people presenting simultaneously with new Type 1 diabetes and Graves' disease.

### Southeast Asians

Fulminant diabetes (a catastrophic illness, usually with history of a few days or a week or two, with a high mortality, and which has some elements of pancreatic exocrine dysfunction) was first described in 2000, and is now commonly reported in Japan and more recently Thailand. Three cases have been described in white French women. It is classified as a form of autoantibody-negative (Type 1B) diabetes. It has not been described so far in the UK. The onset is so rapid that $HbA_{1c}$ levels at presentation are often non-diabetic (i.e. <6.5%, 48 mmol/mol).

## POORLY CONTROLLED PATIENTS WITH KNOWN TYPE 1 DIABETES

Type 1 patients do not usually present to the emergency services unless they are unwell, though most clinics have a handful of patients with 'brittle' diabetes, often associated with neuropathic complications – especially gastroparesis – or eating disorders. They will be known to the emergency department and probably the inpatient diabetes service because of frequent admissions with DKA or hypoglycaemia. Most hospital clinics have quite small numbers of Type 1 patients – perhaps 300–500, and the diabetes team will know many of them personally.

Sometimes they attend because they have run out of insulin supplies. You must make sure that on discharge from the hospital they either have an emergency supply from the pharmacy, or a prescription that can be filled immediately. Type 1 patients can develop DKA if they miss only 1 meal-time injection (**Chapter 1, Figure 8.1**).

A particularly vulnerable group in the UK is Eastern Europeans. Because of uneven care in their home countries, control can be poor, and high rates of smoking and alcohol intake mean that microvascular and macrovascular complications are quite common. They may not be in the primary care system, and can find it difficult to get insulin and other supplies.

- Always assess patients carefully for ketosis or early DKA
- If possible get the inpatient diabetes team to see them promptly
- Additional problems may not be immediately apparent, for example, family conflicts that prevent the patient accessing their insulin supplies at home

## NEWLY PRESENTING TYPE 2 DIABETES

Very common, either self-presentation with symptomatic hyperglycaemia or via referral from general practice because of symptoms or diagnostic glucose levels on routine testing.

### Ethnicity

**Black Africans and African-Caribbeans:** 'Flatbush' diabetes, first described in Brooklyn, New York, in the early 1990s, is increasingly common in the UK:

• Overweight or obese subjects in their 30s or 40s presenting with hyperglycaemia
• Check urinary and capillary ketones and venous blood gas (VBG) – they may have the characteristic DKA of this condition – which requires initial treatment in the usual way
• It is now the commonest form of ketosis-prone diabetes, but is not autoimmune, and patients can usually discontinue insulin treatment a few weeks or months after discharge

**South Asians (India, Pakistan, Bangladesh):**   Most diabetes presenting to emergency departments is Type 2 (broadly speaking, South Asians develop Type 2 diabetes about 10 years before Europeans, therefore in their 30s and 40s). Type 1 diabetes is uncommon, but certainly occurs. Family history, especially in first-degree relatives, is a very strong predictor of Type 2 diabetes.

**South-East Asians:**   Type 2 patients are often slim and insulin requiring, but not ketosis-prone.

### Symptomatic hyperglycaemia

**Osmotic symptoms:**   thirst, urinary frequency, intermittently blurred vision (not corrected by simple refraction).

**Infections:**   staphylococcal skin infections or genital candidal infections.

**Weight loss:**   sometimes acute, but occasionally chronic and very marked – anticipate severe hyperglycaemia and possible HHS in these patients.

Check routine blood tests, especially creatinine and electrolytes, and calculate serum osmolarity. If >320, then this is HHS and admit. If urinary ketones are ≥1+, check capillary ketones. If >1.5 mmol/L, check VBG for pH and $HCO_3$. If <7.3 and <17 respectively, this is DKA (or a mixed picture if osmolarity >320).

### Ensure adequate follow-up

If there is uncomplicated hyperglycaemia, discharge. But ensure:

• Rapid follow-up with general practice team
• Ensure that you start treatment: e.g. metformin 500 mg bd if no contraindications, together with a low dose of a sulphonylurea, e.g. gliclazide 40 mg bd to ensure symptoms come under rapid control (warn about mid-morning hypoglycaemia)

## PATIENTS ATTENDING THE ED WITH HIGH BLOOD GLUCOSE LEVELS

### Management of high blood glucose levels in patients who do not require admission

If there is severe hyperglycaemia but no DKA or HHS – think twice before discharging patients who present with BG levels >25 mmol/L.

There is no 'danger' BG threshold that demands admission. Random glucose levels of 20–25 mmol/L are frequent events in otherwise well patients, especially Type 1 (**Figure 8.2**). In Type 1 patients very high BG levels may be a physiological and eating response to hypoglycaemia up to 6–12 hours before. However, if BG is >25, and especially near 30 or above be cautious about discharging a patient, even if there is no overt DKA or HHS:

- There may be a serious underlying medical problem
- It may be early HHS
- It may be early DKA
- Patients are likely to have osmotic symptoms (thirst, polyuria) at these levels
- If it's associated with high HbA$_{1c}$ (look it up if you can) then the patient will need treatment intensifying – though not necessarily as an inpatient
- Type 1 patients usually don't present to ED unless in DKA or severe hypoglycaemia. If there is a specialist team available, they are likely to know the patient. Contact them. If they aren't around, leave a message for them

Exclude a concomitant medical problem, start VRIII and i.v. rehydration. Assess after 4–6 hours. If BG has not significantly fallen, then there is probably something going on that isn't obvious and that requires formal diagnosis. Admit.

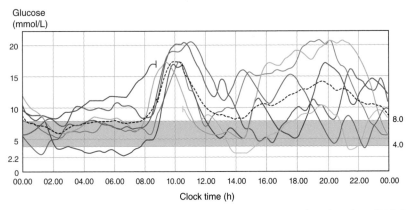

**Figure 8.2** Continuous subcutaneous (interstitial) glucose monitoring (CGM) tracings (iPRO 2, Medtronic) over 6 days in a Type 1 patient (using an insulin pump, though not very satisfactorily). Note the prolonged hypoglycaemia on one night, the frequent BG peaks up to 20 mmol/L and the consistent major glycaemic peaks after breakfast. This is a very common finding in both Type 1 and Type 2 diabetes, even when there is no preceding hypoglycaemia. The dawn phenomenon is often blamed (rising BG levels in the hours before waking resulting from surges in growth hormone levels, which does not seem to be the problem in this case), but another major contribution may be the very high glycaemic index of most breakfast cereals.

### If patient can be discharged – it is your responsibility to ensure that the patient is adequately followed up

- Precise prescription
- Sufficient medication/insulin and home blood glucose monitoring equipment to last until the next encounter with HCP (prescribe insulin pens and cartridges in multiples of 5; packs contain 5 items and cannot be split).

- Clear arrangements for follow-up:
  - Type 1 patients need specialist follow-up (consultant, specialist registrar or diabetes nurse specialist)
  - Type 2 patients can be referred back to primary care, but arrangements must be secure (written, email, etc.)

**Type 1 patients and insulin-treated Type 2 patients**
Ensure insulin regimen is broadly appropriate:

- Day and night are covered with insulin preparations that last sufficiently long (e.g. reinstate fast-acting breakfast dose – and breakfast – if previously omitted. Start with 4 units)
- If there is any consistent pattern to hyperglycaemia increase the previous dose(s) by 10%
- Remind patients of targets for Type 1 diabetes: fasting BG 5–8, postprandial <10 mmol/L
- Brief education in self-titration: increase doses by 1 or 2 units (no more than that) every 3 or 4 days

**Type 2 patients**
Increase medication, but in the emergency setting limit the repertoire to metformin and sulphonylurea. Examples:

- Increase metformin to maximum effective dose, i.e. 2 g daily (1 g bd)
- Increase sulphonylurea, e.g. gliclazide to 80 mg bd (higher doses are probably not effective)
- If patient is taking metformin only, then add sulphonylurea, e.g. gliclazide 40 mg bd (but warn about symptoms of hypoglycaemia, characteristically 3–4 hours after dose)

# 9 Diabetic ketoacidosis

## Give soluble insulin intravenously at 6 U/hr

**Key points**

- The problem is insulin deficiency, *not* hyperglycaemia
- Make the diagnosis carefully
- Although DKA is a medical emergency, it is rarely life-threatening, and 'aggressive' treatment (with very large amounts of fluid and indiscriminate insulin) can be harmful, especially in the young and elderly, where it can cause cerebral oedema and fluid overload, respectively
- Priorities: correct the acidosis, replace fluid and give insulin primarily to suppress ketogenesis and only secondarily to reduce blood glucose
- Aim to discharge patients with uncomplicated DKA within 24 hours (an aim, though, not a target)

## CONFIRM THE DIAGNOSIS

Because there is a specific and intensive 'protocol' associated with the management of DKA, it's critical to make the diagnosis precisely. All the following are needed (**Table 9.1**):

- **Diabetes**
- **Ketosis**
- **Acidosis**

**Table 9.1** The working biochemical diagnosis of DKA

| Hyperglycaemia | 'Officially' BG >14 mmol/L (USA) | Usually >20, rarely >30–40 (consider mixed DKA/HHS) |
|---|---|---|
| Ketosis | • Urinary ketones ≥2+ (>3.9 mmol/L) <br> • Capillary ketones, usually >4 mmol/L | |
| Acidosis <br> Venous bicarbonate | Venous pH <7.3 <br> ≤17 mmol/L | Severe and high risk if <7.0 <br> In the early compensated phase, bicarbonate buffers ketoacids, so bicarbonate is low but pH normal |

*The Hands-on Guide to Diabetes Care in Hospital,* First Edition by David Levy.
© 2016 John Wiley & Sons, Ltd. Published 2016 by John Wiley & Sons, Ltd.

Remember there is a differential diagnosis (that is, other causes of metabolic acidosis and of ketosis), and also a spectrum of diabetes that does not always amount to full-blown DKA (**Chapter 8**; **Figure 9.1**).

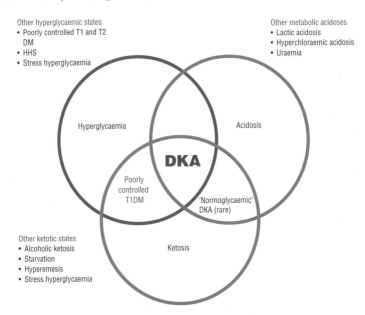

Other hyperglycaemic states
• Poorly controlled T1 and T2 DM
• HHS
• Stress hyperglycaemia

Other metabolic acidoses
• Lactic acidosis
• Hyperchloraemic acidosis
• Uraemia

Hyperglycaemia

Acidosis

**DKA**

Poorly controlled T1DM

'Normoglycaemic' DKA (rare)

Other ketotic states
• Alcoholic ketosis
• Starvation
• Hyperemesis
• Stress hyperglycaemia

Ketosis

**Figure 9.1** The differential diagnosis of DKA, and the spectrum of diabetes that is out of control without being DKA. (Adapted from Fisher JN, Kitabchi AE. A randomized study of phosphate therapy in the treatment of diabetic ketoacidosis. *J Clin Endocrinol Metab* 1983; 57: 177–180.)

## INDICATORS OF SEVERITY (Table 9.2)

**Table 9.2** Features of severity. ICU outreach teams are adept at dealing with shocked patients (of course), but contact them urgently if you are seeing a sick patient with severe metabolic disturbance or its associations

|  | Significance | Action |
| --- | --- | --- |
| **Clinical** | | |
| Indicators of shock | | Urgent ICU referral |
| Kussmaul respiration | Likely severe metabolic acidosis | ICU assessment |
| Impairment of conscious level | Likely severe metabolic derangement (cerebral oedema or other intracranial diagnosis) | Consider brain CT: ICU assessment |
| Abdominal pain | Likely severe metabolic acidosis | Surgical assessment |
| **Laboratory** | | |
| Osmolarity >320 | Possible mixed DKA/HHS | Urgent ICU referral |
| pH <7.0 | | May be resistant |
| Leucocytosis >25 | Likely significant infection | Full infection screen (temp may be normal or low) |
| Elevated amylase | Correlates with pH and osmolarity | |

## OVERALL MANAGEMENT PRIORITIES

### Where should the patient be managed?

**Routine cases** — acute admissions unit or diabetes/endocrine/metabolism ward

Most cases of DKA, for example, precipitated by a simple infection, insulin omission, acute alcohol excess or viral GI upset, will resolve within 24 hours. These patients should be managed in an area experienced in dealing with hyperglycaemic emergencies, either an acute admissions unit or diabetes ward, preferably with facilities for measuring capillary blood ketones. Non-medical wards where nursing staff are not experienced in managing these cases are not the right place.

**Complex cases** — ICU   Few patients require immediate ICU attention, but if metabolic correction is slower than outlined in **Table 9.3**, ask ICU to assess the patient sooner rather than later.

**Table 9.3** The usual trajectory of patients with uncomplicated DKA

| | Target | Aim time to correct | Measurement frequency/ comment |
|---|---|---|---|
| **Correct acidosis** | >7.3 | Within 4 hours | Hourly venous gases until ≥7.3 |
| **Correct ketosis** | Capillary ketones <1 mmol/L | Within 12 hours | 4-hourly capillary ketones |
| **Establish reasonable BG levels** | BG levels 5–15 | Within 24 hours | Hourly until acidosis and ketosis corrected; thereafter 2–4 hourly |
| **Establish cause** | | As soon as possible | Detailed history, especially if recurrent DKA |
| **Discharge** | All above, plus establishing antihyperglycaemic regimen | Within 24 hours | |

### Immediate to-dos

- Capillary glucose, capillary ketones, venous gases
- i.v. line running 0.9% NaCl[1] 1 L over 1 hour (only start NaCl with KCl when you know [$K^+$] to be <5.5 mmol/L – venous gas measurement is sufficiently accurate initially)
- Routine blood tests:
  - Creatinine and electrolytes, FBC, CRP
  - Phosphate, magnesium, CK, amylase in sick patients
  - Lipaemic sample: implies severe metabolic disturbance, amylase measurement may be unreliable, and the laboratory won't be able to do other serum measurements (e.g. LFTs)
- Urinalysis for ketones and infection

---

[1] Current recommendations are to use 0.9% NaCl in hyperglycaemic emergencies, despite its hypertonicity ([$Na^+$] = 154 mmol/L). PlasmaLyte 148 would be preferable ([$Na^+$] = 140 mmol/L), but it contains a fixed low [$K^+$] = 5 mmol/L, and much higher KCl concentrations are needed in DKA, where potassium depletion is likely to be severe.

**Then**

- Start i.v. insulin infusion (50 units soluble or rapid-acting analogue insulin, nearly always Actrapid (soluble insulin [Novo Nordisk]) in the UK in 50 mL syringe pump, running at 6 mL(U)/hr[2]
- Chest X ray
- 12 lead ECG
- If shock or impaired consciousness, call ICU team and place urinary catheter

## ASK THE FOLLOWING AFTER DIAGNOSIS, INITIAL ASSESSMENT AND IMMEDIATE TREATMENT

**Have another think about the severity of the case: does the patient require ICU assessment?**

May do if any of these are present:

- Shocked (very unusual)
- Impaired level of consciousness (impairment is related to degree of metabolic derangement)
- Kussmaul respiration (related to degree of acidosis)
- Abdominal pain (related to degree of acidosis)
- pH: severe DKA if <7.0 (moderate 7.00-7.24; mild 7.25-7.30)

**Are there any other medical or surgical problems that might complicate management?**

- Alcohol or drugs
- Other causes of abdominal pain (pancreatitis – consider if serum is lipaemic)
- Infection (chest, urinary tract, gastrointestinal, foot)

**Is the inpatient diabetes team available to help with the management?**

**If patient does not need intensive care, can you ensure that the patient is cared for in an appropriate clinical environment (this usually means an acute admission unit for the first 12 hours at least)?**

**Complete any 'routine' investigations**

- ECG
- Chest X ray
- Brain CT if impaired level of consciousness

**Prescriptions**

- Write up venous thromboprophylaxis; consider full anticoagulation if there is associated hyperosmolarity (>320 mOsmol/L) and no contraindications
- Ensure any long-acting insulin (Lantus, Levemir, Humulin I, Insuman Basal, Tresiba – **Chapter 20**) is written up in the usual dose to be given at the usual time (if the previous day's dose was forgotten, give a proportionate amount; omit if the next routine dose is too close – for example less than 6 hours)

---

[2] There is controversy about the rate of insulin infusion, but the controversy does not have a sound clinical evidence base. Theoretically ketosis is suppressed optimally at 0.1 U/kg/hr. In practice, a fixed rate of 6 U/hr works well, it is difficult to estimate weight accurately in sick people in the emergency department, and there is potential for error in prescription. Most hospitals use 6 U/hr, as it is easy to remember and works.

## Additional history

While waiting for the results of the initial investigations to come through, take a more detailed history, focusing on the cause of the episode:

- Infection (30–40% of cases, most commonly GI)
- Omitting insulin (15–30%)
  - Failure to observe sick-day rule to continue insulin even when ill (**Chapter 30**)
  - Running out of insulin supplies
  - Common in youngsters: partying with alcohol ± vomiting and omitting overnight basal insulin
- Drugs (especially cocaine)
- 'Brittle diabetes': recurrent DKA mostly in young women with unstable diabetes
- Young women with disordered eating and associated insulin omission
- Patients with advanced renal failure, often with recurrent infections and foot ulceration
- Gastroparesis
- Reports of DKA with modestly elevated glucose levels in Type 2 patients taking SGLT-2 inhibitor drugs ('flozins'; **Chapter 24**), precipitated by major illness, reduced food and fluid intake and reduced insulin dose

## ACUTE MANAGEMENT — UP TO 4 HOURS

### Aim to normalise pH in 4 hours

- Key treatment: patients should be on their 3rd litre of 0.9% NaCl by 4 hours
- Hourly VBG until pH ≥7.3
- pH will usually normalise after 4–6 hours. If pH is not rising, intensify fluid replacement (0.9% 1L 1–2 hourly). Use [K$^+$] levels from VBG to guide KCl replacement (40 mmol with each litre of fluid, so long as [K$^+$] <5.5 mmol/L)
- Sodium bicarbonate probably does not help but intensivists may suggest one bolus of 1.26% NaHCO$_3^-$ if pH isn't rising (500 mL over 30 minutes)
- If pH is not rising above 7.0, ask ICU team to see urgently. Severe dehydration and tissue hypoxia with resistant acidosis is a problem in some patients, and they may respond rapidly to acute haemofiltration for 4–12 hours

### Correct ketosis – should begin to reduce within 4 hours

Four-hourly capillary ketones until <1.0 mmol/L

### Fluids – hyperacute, then acute replacement

Continue 0.9% NaCl.[3] Aim to replace fluid as follows:

### DURATION OF EACH LITRE OF 0.9% NACL:

Initially 1 hour, then 2 hours, 2, 4, 4 and 6–8 hours

## MANAGEMENT FROM 4–12 HOURS

### Triple infusion once blood glucose <14 mmol/L

Patients need continuing rehydration and continuing 6 U/hr insulin to suppress ketosis.
   They therefore need higher concentration glucose to prevent hypoglycaemia, once BG levels have fallen.

---

[3] There are potential risks of using high volumes of NaCl, including transient hyperchloraemic acidosis.

UK recommendation is to use a triple infusion regimen until ketosis has resolved:

- Continuing fluid replacement (0.9% NaCl)
- Continuing insulin at 6 U/hr
- 10% glucose at 125 mL/hr (500 mL 4 hourly)

These fluids are all compatible, and ingenious piggy-backing of infusions and lines means that patients do not need to suffer the discomfort of two separate i.v. lines delivered to them (**Figure 9.2**).

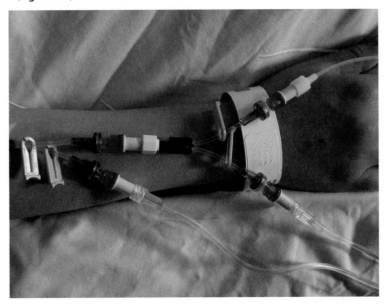

**Figure 9.2** Triple infusion running in a patient with DKA. All three (glucose, rehydrating fluid and insulin) can be safely given through a single cannula.

### Check electrolytes at 8 hours
- Focus on [Na$^+$] (not usually a problem in DKA unless there is associated hyperosmolarity and risk of hypernatraemia – >145 mmol/L)
- Low [K$^+$], often in the range 3.0–3.5 mmol/L, is common, and caused by a combination of insulin driving potassium into cells, resolution of acidosis and failure to appreciate the severe total body potassium deficit. Correct with i.v. KCl (40 mmol with each litre of fluid) so long as renal function is normal
- Don't write up fluids beyond the next 6 hours – you don't know what the electrolytes will show

### Eating and drinking
If there is no major underlying medical cause for the DKA, patients will often be eating and drinking at this stage. If so, restart their usual insulin regimen, and discontinue rehydrating fluids if electrolytes are normal. But ketosis can be slow to resolve; most patients will need high dose i.v. insulin and glucose for 24 hours.

If ketosis has resolved, but the patient is not eating and drinking, then change to a standard VRIII with 5% glucose until they are eating and drinking.

## MANAGEMENT FROM 12–24 HOURS

Most patients will be eating and drinking, ketone-free and anxious to go home after 24 hours, but ketosis may persist. Remember that urinary ketones persist after serum β-OH butyrate has fallen to undetectable levels. Ketosis signifies insulin deficiency, and if capillary ketones are still >1.0 mmol/L after everything else has resolved, then there is an undiagnosed medical problem – usually infection, but DKA complicated by or precipitated by alcohol (acute or chronic use) can prolong the ketosis. Don't discharge the patient, however well they are, until you have made the diagnosis (or you can discharge the patient with a meter to monitor capillary ketones every 12 hours until resolution).

## PLANNING FOR DISCHARGE

Average length of stay for DKA is 24–48 hours.

Ensure diabetes specialist nurses/inpatient diabetes team have reviewed the patient, and have made firm arrangements for follow up within 24–48 hours (this can be by telephone).

If the inpatient team isn't around (weekend, public holiday. etc.) get a brief senior review to ensure the patient is well for discharge, and communicate with the inpatient team when they return – email if possible. Give the patient their contact details.

*Newly diagnosed Type 1 patients admitted over a weekend* need intensive education during their index admission. In hospitals where there is specialist 7-day cover, there is no problem, but many will need to remain in hospital until they can be seen first thing when the diabetes inpatient nursing team returns. Pressure to discharge patients must be resisted until they are confident dealing with this major and lifelong condition; you won't recall, but only 25 years ago most patients with new-onset Type 1 diabetes (presenting with DKA or otherwise) would be admitted for 1–2 weeks to 'stabilise' their diabetes.

**Box 9.1** shows a simple checklist for discharge.

---

**Box 9.1**   Checklist for discharge of DKA patients

- Sufficient insulin (or a prescription that can be immediately filled) until the patient can get further supplies from their primary care team. Use the table in **Chapter 23** for substitute insulin preparations suitable for short-term use. The differences in practice between insulin preparations in the same class are small. Reassure the patient, but remind them that the onset and offset of action may be different
- Home blood glucose monitoring (HBGM) equipment (strips, lancets, monitoring book where they can write BG results)
- Insulin needles (5-mm length, 4 mm in very slim people)
- Brief education about symptoms of hypoglycaemia (tremor, palpitations, anxiety, sweating, hunger, pins and needles)
- Make sure they carry fast-acting carbohydrate with them (glucose tablets, snack-size chocolate bars)
- Patients can drive so long as they are medically well, their vision is unaffected (osmotic lens effects with blurring and difficulty in focusing are common) and they have been fully educated in recognition and management of hypoglycaemia. However, they should drive as little as possible until they have had much more complete education. Newly diagnosed patients should contact the DVLA to let them know about the new diagnosis

# Further reading

Joint British Diabetes Societies for Inpatient Care Guideline. The management of diabetic ketoacidosis in adults (revised September 2013). Available from: www.diabetologists-abcd.org.uk/JBDS/JBDS.htm (accessed on 26 March 2015).

Kamel KS, Halperin ML. Acid–base problems in diabetic ketoacidosis. *N Engl J Med*. 2015;372:546–54. PMID: 25651248.

Kitabchi AE, Fisher JN. Diabetes mellitus. In: Glew RA, Peters SP (eds). Clinical studies in medical biochemistry. New York: Oxford University Press; 1987. p. 105.

**See Chapter 34 for a DKA aide-memoire.**

# 10 Hyperosmolar hyperglycaemic state (HHS)

**Top tip**

More difficult to manage than DKA, and has a higher morbidity and mortality. Insulin is less of a priority than in DKA, despite the often severe hyperglycaemia. Use low-dose insulin and gentler fluid replacement in these patients who are usually older and with comorbidities.

## Initially give soluble insulin intravenously at 2U/hr

**Key points**

- About 50% of cases are new presentations of Type 2 diabetes. Non-specific symptoms are common (e.g. increasing drowsiness, reluctance to eat and drink)
- Be precise in making the diagnosis (even though there is no official definition): always calculate osmolarity
- Can coexist with DKA
- Priorities: correct the fluid deficit, watch renal function carefully, gently reduce the often very high glucose levels with low-dose insulin
- Once resolved, think carefully about the treatment needed

## CONFIRM THE DIAGNOSIS (Table 10.1)

Table 10.1 The key positive and negative laboratory features of the hyperosmolar state

| | | |
|---|---|---|
| **Hyperosmolarity** | >320 mOsmol/kg (severe >340) Calculate: $2\times[Na^+] + [urea] + [glucose]$ | $[K^+]$ (officially $2\times [K^+]$) is too small to make a clinically significant difference to the result |
| **Hyperglycaemia** | No official criterion level, but usually >30 mmol/L, frequently ~50, and occasionally as high as 100+ | High BG probably contributes most to the hyperviscosity which drives the high thromboembolic risk |
| **Lack of acidosis (unless mixed DKA/HHS picture)** | Venous pH >7.3 Bicarbonate >18 mmol/L | Always check VBG |
| **Lack of ketosis (unless mixed picture)** | Allow up to 1+ urinary ketones for starvation, but capillary ketones should be <1 mmol/L | Always check capillary blood ketones |

*The Hands-on Guide to Diabetes Care in Hospital,* First Edition by David Levy.
© 2016 John Wiley & Sons, Ltd. Published 2016 by John Wiley & Sons, Ltd.

## INDICATORS OF SEVERITY (Table 10.2)

Table 10.2 Indicators of severity in HHS. Ask for early ICU assessment in all sick patients

| Clinical | Significance | Action |
|---|---|---|
| Indicators of shock | | Request urgent ICU assessment |
| Any impairment of conscious level | Likely severe metabolic derangement (decreasing GCS with increasing osmolarity >325–330) But high comorbidity, so think about stroke, drug effects | Drowsiness or worse: ask for ICU assessment |
| 'Package' of adverse prognostic features: • Serum Cr >300 • Osmolarity >340 • Low GCS, e.g. 6 or lower • Low urine output • Acidosis (CKD, metformin, sepsis) | Greater risk of early mortality | Extreme vigilance and multidisciplinary input at an early stage (acute physicians, diabetes team, ICU) |
| Associated infection | Renal tract, chest, skin, foot | |
| Hypernatraemia [Na$^+$] >145 after correction for prevailing plasma glucose | Absolute hypernatraemia is a risk for osmotic demyelination; rapid reduction (e.g. >8–12 mmol/24 hr) is also a risk | Cautious fluid replacement in all cases; calculate corrected [Na$^+$] frequently |

## MANAGEMENT PRIORITIES (Table 10.3)

Table 10.3 Management priorities in HHS. HHS rarely resolves as quickly as DKA on account of the age of the patients and their comorbidities

| | Target | Target time to correct | Measurement frequency |
|---|---|---|---|
| **Osmolarity** | <300 mOsmol/kg | 24–48 hours | Calculate 8-hourly |
| **Serum [Na$^+$]** | <140 mmol/L | Depending on initial corrected [Na$^+$]: no faster than 8–12 mmol/24 hr | 8-hourly |
| **Glucose** | 10–15 mmol/L | 24 hours: ideally no faster than 2–3 mmol/hr, especially if very high to begin with | Hourly when in meter range |
| **Renal function** | Back to baseline | Variable, but often rapid. Often does not settle completely to pre-admission levels, especially if previously impaired | 8-hourly |

### Immediate to-dos

- Capillary glucose (mandatory laboratory glucose if CBG above the meter limit (e.g. 28–33 mmol/L – if you don't have an accurate glucose value, you can't determine osmolarity, and therefore you can't make the diagnosis)

- Capillary ketones, venous blood gases
- i.v. line running 0.9% NaCl 1 L over 1 hour (many patients will have high [$K^+$] as a result of CKD/AKI ± angiotensin blockade treatment with ACE-i/ARB, so don't give KCl until you have a laboratory measurement (venous gas result is sufficiently accurate to gauge whether or not to start potassium replacement)
- Routine blood tests: if you take the blood yourself, note whether it is 'thick' – implies very high glucose and osmolarity and high thrombosis risk. If lipaemic, consider pancreatitis
- If obviously sick, add troponin, magnesium, CK and amylase
- Ask for ICU advice if low GCS – suggests severe metabolic derangement
- Don't start insulin immediately, and definitely NOT at 6 or more U/hr – non-insulin-mediated glucose (i.e. renal) disposal will cause glucose level to fall with rehydration. Most guidelines suggest delaying insulin for 1–2 hours, some practitioners suggest as long as 12 hours
- Strongly discourage emergency department staff from 'aggressive' treatment, for example, very high doses of i.v. insulin, 'stat' litres of fluid: these can result in major osmotic shifts, especially harmful to the brain

**Then**

- Chest X ray
- 12 lead ECG
- Brief clinical examination: focus on GCS, volume status, infection (especially feet, chest and urine)
- Urinary catheter if impaired conscious level

## CORRECTING SERUM [$Na^+$] FOR PREVAILING GLUCOSE

True hypernatraemia can be disguised by severe hyperglycaemia, which depresses serum [$Na^+$]. This is common in HHS, where BG levels are especially high. In the early stages of managing HHS, request simultaneous laboratory glucose and electrolytes, and correct laboratory [$Na^+$] using the formula:

**True [$Na^+$] = laboratory [$Na^+$] + [glucose (mmol/)/4]**

If corrected [$Na^+$] is rising towards 150 mmol/L, then carefully monitored alternating litres of 0.45% ('half-normal') saline with either 0.9% saline or PlasmaLyte 148 should limit the rise in serum [$Na^+$]

- Discuss with a senior before prescribing hypotonic solutions

## ASK THE FOLLOWING AFTER DIAGNOSIS, INITIAL ASSESSMENT AND TREATMENT

**Does this patient need, or are they likely to soon need, intensive care?**
HHS patients are likely to have severe renal impairment, sepsis, poor organ perfusion and impaired left ventricular function that may require inotropic support, meticulous fluid balance and possibly dialysis. Patients with mixed acidosis and hyperosmolarity must be assessed by intensivists. Always err on the side of caution in requesting ICU input.

**Is the inpatient diabetes team around to help with the management?**

**If the patient does not need intensive care, can you ensure that they are looked after in a suitably staffed and equipped environment?**

This will mean an acute admission unit in most cases; patients should not be transferred to a general medical ward for at least 24 hours, or until vital signs normalise, and renal function begins to improve.

## COMPLETE ANY 'ROUTINE' INVESTIGATIONS

- ECG
- Chest X ray
- Brain CT if impaired level of consciousness

## ADDITIONAL HISTORY

Important, but may not be available from the patient. Focus on:

- Ambulance record (if available): was the patient found lying on the floor (risk of rhabdomyolysis)?
- Is the patient known to have diabetes?
- If known diabetes, is there a history of impaired cognition (risk of omitting medication and insulin)?
- Medication: high-dose glucocorticoids the likeliest culprit, but both HHS and DKA are well-recognised in association with atypical antipsychotic agents, especially olanzapine, risperidone and to a lesser extent quetiapine, usually in patients with known diabetes

## PRESCRIPTIONS

- Write up venous thromboprophylaxis. Patients with associated hyperosmolarity (>320 mOsmol/kg) should have full anticoagulation after appropriate risk assessment. If severe (>340 mOsmol/kg) there is a very high risk of venous or arterial thrombosis
- Discontinue oral hypoglycaemic agents, especially metformin (usually severely impaired renal function) and gliptins and GLP-1 analogues (risk of acute pancreatitis)
- Discontinue angiotensin blocking agents and statins

## CONTINUING MANAGEMENT UP TO 24–48 HOURS

- Stabilise BP if necessary and ensure urine output is satisfactory
- Continue gentle correction of biochemistry
- No worsening of corrected [Na$^+$]
- No worsening of level of consciousness

If it feels like the overall clinical situation is worsening (see **Table 10.2**), ask ICU for advice.

### Fluids
Conventionally 0.9% NaCl is used, unless there is impending or actual hypernatraemia (corrected [Na$^+$] >145 mmol/L). Fluid replacement should be guided by the clinical state, but this is a rough guide:

### DURATION OF EACH LITRE OF 0.9% NACL:
Initially 1 hour, then 2 hours, 4, 4, 6, 6, 8 hours

### Insulin
- Increase rate by 1–2 U/hr if BG levels are not falling gently (e.g. 3 mmol/L/hr)

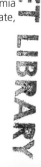

- Do not use high dose insulin (6 U/hr) – there is no ketosis to suppress, and rapid falls in glucose will contribute to rapid falls in [Na⁺]
- Once BG is stabilised at 10–14 mmol/L, use low fixed-dose insulin if it holds BG levels steady, or start a standard VRIII if unstable, or the patient has started eating. It is probably best to keep i.v. insulin running until biochemistry has stabilised

## CONTINUING MANAGEMENT — USUALLY AFTER 24 HOURS

### Patients who will require long-term insulin treatment:

*Previously insulin-treated patients*: the regimen may need intensifying, for example, twice-daily biphasic if previously taking basal insulin, basal-bolus regimen if previously taking biphasic insulin. Non-insulin agents can continue, but they will probably have little effect (withdraw or reduce metformin according to where eGFR settles; see **Chapter 24**).

*Patients previously treated with non-insulin agents*: this is a difficult clinical situation, and you will need advice from the diabetes team. HHS is a very severe hyperglycaemic state, so it is unlikely that pre-admission treatment will be sufficient – unless the admission was precipitated by not taking medication over a prolonged period, for example, more than a few weeks (this is not uncommon).

### Insulin treatment is safer where:

- there is ketosis with hyperosmolarity
- there is evidence of gradual deterioration in control over years
- there has been significant weight loss, especially if the patient is not currently overweight (suggests progressive insulin deficiency)
- there is very poor control (A1C >9%, 75 mmol/mol) on maximum non-insulin agents and good compliance
- steroids precipitated the HHS (**see Chapter 29**)
- there has been poor compliance with medication before admission, and once-daily insulin could be more reliably given by carers, relatives or community nurses

### Newly presenting patients with clear-cut Type 2 diabetes

The temptation is to use metformin alone – and many of these patients will eventually be well-controlled on diet measures and metformin. But metformin does not work quickly enough and titration may take 2–3 months from an initial dose of 500 mg twice daily to the recommended maximum of 1 g twice daily. The only class of non-insulin agents that will work within a few days to lower BG levels is the sulphonylureas (they have the immediate effect of stimulating β-cell secretion of insulin). Gliclazide is the most commonly-used SU in the UK. So prescribe:

- Metformin 500 mg bd
- Gliclazide 40 mg bd
- Both to be taken with breakfast and evening meal

### Advise patients:

**Metformin:**　May upset GI tract in the first week – indigestion, acid reflux, diarrhoea, abdominal pain.

**Gliclazide:**   Have a carbohydrate-containing breakfast (e.g. cereal, 2 slices of bread), and advise a mid-morning snack and to carry glucose in the first few days (peak risk of hypoglycaemia with sulphonylureas is about 4 hours after dosing). Don't omit evening meal.

There is no need for BG self-monitoring at this stage; moderate glycaemic control (e.g. up to 15 mmol/L) without symptomatic hypoglycaemia is the key safety concern immediately after discharge.

Ensure there is a competent diabetes review within a week of discharge (DSNs will advise on the local arrangements, which vary widely). Most patients with straightforward HHS should be reviewed by their primary care team, and will take over their care.

### Anticoagulation

There are no long-term follow up studies of patients admitted with severe hyperosmolarity (>340 mOsmol/kg), but the tendency to thrombosis – venous and arterial – probably continues for several weeks after discharge. Discuss the possibility of a month of full-dose s.c. enoxaparin with the diabetes team and the patient, then re-start low-dose aspirin (unless there are contraindications).

### Historical note

The hyperosmolar state in diabetes was not described until the 1970s (at a time when even the distinction between Type 1 and Type 2 diabetes was unclear). There is very little trial-based evidence for the best way to treat HHS (especially insulin dosing and fluid replacement), and guidance and practice are mostly based on supposition about its causes, and a gradual evolution of best-practice consensus. There are many variants of the details in this section, some of them (understandably) vigorously promoted by teams who may have experienced a poor outcome. Until we have the gold-standard RCT (which hasn't arrived after 40 years, so we shouldn't expect it any time soon), the guiding principles of management are: frequent clinical and biochemical assessment by experienced doctors and nurses in a clinical environment where these complex and sick patients have been managed on many occasions in the past, and gentle correction of the often severe biochemical abnormalities. In this situation, do not make awful numbers worse by 'aggressive' treatments.

### Further reading

Joint British Diabetes Societies for Inpatient Care Guideline. Management of the hyperosmolar hyperglycaemic state (HHS) in adults with diabetes (August 2012). Available from: www.diabetologists-abcd.org.uk/JBDS/JBDS.htm (accessed on 26 March 2015).

**See Chapter 34 for an HHS aide-memoire.**

# 11 Managing acute hypoglycaemia in the emergency department

**(See also Chapters 24 and 26)**

## Top tip

Most hypoglycaemia is self-managed or managed by ambulance personnel. Only patients with severe hypoglycaemia will be seen in the emergency department. Treat it seriously.

## Key points

- Ensure CBG is measured in every patient with impaired consciousness, even if there is another obvious cause. Someone with a stroke may well have diabetes treated with insulin, a sulphonylurea, or both
- Hypoglycaemia is common in people with very poorly controlled diabetes (Type 1 or 2). Insulin-treated Type 2 patients and Type 1 patients have the same frequency of severe hypoglycaemia
- Injuries sustained while hypoglycaemic are common
- Don't discharge patients until you have adjusted their treatment and ensured they are returning to a safe environment
- If the diabetes team is in the hospital, ask them to see the patient. They are likely to know useful details about patients, especially if they have recurrent hypoglycaemia or 'brittle' Type 1 diabetes

## Unusual presentations of hypoglycaemia
- Seizure
- Hemiparesis
- Aggressive (possibly criminal) behaviour
- 'He's been drinking, doctor'
- Acute back pain (opisthotonos or rarely crush fracture of thoracic vertebra caused by fitting)

## TREATMENT (see Chapter 26)

Blood glucose levels may already be high after treatment when the patient arrives at the hospital. Read the ambulance or paramedic records, noting CBG levels and clock times. Don't compound the problem by illogically setting up an insulin infusion (VRIII) to

*The Hands-on Guide to Diabetes Care in Hospital,* First Edition by David Levy.
© 2016 John Wiley & Sons, Ltd. Published 2016 by John Wiley & Sons, Ltd.

correct the high blood glucose levels (late recurrent hypoglycaemia with long-acting insulin preparations or sulphonylureas is the obvious risk). You might be surprised how often this is done.

### Sulphonylurea-induced hypoglycaemia (see Chapter 24)

Most sulphonylureas are long-acting, so admit all patients with sulphonylurea-induced hypoglycaemia. The peak effect of sulphonylureas is at 4–8 hours, so the commonest time for acute hypoglycaemia is late morning (though in inpatients the peak time is the early hours of the morning). The usual scenario is an older, thin person who may have lost more weight recently for a variety of reasons, and is either very careful with their diet or whose appetite has gone down. They usually have low or very low $HbA_{1c}$ (e.g. 5–6.5%, 31–48 mmol/mol).

Avoid glucagon, as it may stimulate residual insulin secretion and make the hypoglycaemia worse. After the acute treatment, start a 10% i.v. glucose infusion, initially at 100 mL/hr, measure CBG hourly, and maintain for at least 12 hours. If there is recurrent severe hypoglycaemia despite i.v. glucose, give the somatostatin analogue octreotide, which inhibits insulin and glucagon secretion (as well as many other hormones) – 50 mcg s.c. 12-hourly.

### When to admit

- Patients with sulphonylurea-induced hypoglycaemia
- Patients with residual neurological deficits or prolonged coma after treatment: consider postictal state, cerebral oedema, head injury, intracranial infection, bleed or infarction, and coexisting poisoning with alcohol or drugs. Get an urgent brain CT scan
- Patients living on their own with no facilities for close supervision over the next 24 hours. In Type 1 diabetes, episodes of severe hypoglycaemia tend to cluster. One factor is probably further impairment of hypoglycaemia awareness following the first episode
- Recurrent hypoglycaemia after successful initial treatment (liver disease, overdose with long-acting insulin or sulphonylurea, intentional or otherwise)
- Remember non-diabetic causes of hypoglycaemia, and take blood for insulin and C-peptide if CBG <2.5 mmol/L

### Follow-up

- Ensure your patient has food after recovery. Replenish depleted hepatic glycogen stores with a substantial carbohydrate-containing snack (e.g. 3–6 biscuits, bread, or sandwiches)
- Check CBG after 20 minutes
- If the patient has recovered, is fully conscious and has a blood glucose >7 mmol/L within an hour, they can be discharged (so long as they will not be on their own).-
- *Driving*: attendance at an emergency department with hypoglycaemia (including nocturnal hypoglycaemia) is a reportable event. The current UK rules are:
  - Group 1 driver (car/motorcycle) who has had two or more assistance-requiring hypoglycaemic episodes in the past 12 months must inform the DVLA, and be advised not to drive
  - Group 2 driver (bus/lorry) who has had one or more episodes in the past 12 months must do likewise

- If the diabetes team cannot see the patient on this admission:
  - Target the culprit insulin dose if possible and reduce by 20%. If it's not clear which dose was at fault or a recent HbA$_{1c}$ is low (e.g. <7%, 53 mmol/mol), reduce all insulin doses by 10%. Halve the dose of sulphonylurea or discontinue
  - Make firm arrangements for prompt follow-up. No vagueries, please: 'the diabetes team will get in touch' [presumably through telepathy], 'go and see your GP', 'we'll write to your GP', etc.
  - Take the patient's or carer's contact details
  - Write, email or leave voicemail message with the diabetes team

# PART 3
# Acute medical and surgical problems commonly complicated by diabetes

# 12 Presentation of cardiac disease in diabetic patients

**Top tip**

Always consider acute coronary syndrome (ACS) in any diabetic patient, Type 1 or 2, presenting with vague upper body discomfort.

## FEATURES OF ACS (Box 12.1)

**Box 12.1**

- Atypical chest symptoms are very common in diabetes, and according to the clinical picture, you will need to think of ACS, heart failure and pulmonary embolism
- Groups at particular risk of ACS include younger women (Type 1 and Type 2), ethnic minority men, patients with longstanding Type 1 diabetes, and renal patients (diabetic nephropathy and dialysis)
- Diffuse and extensive coronary disease is common, and invasive strategies carry better outcomes (see **Chapter 12**). Ask for cardiac opinion, discuss and refer early

Classical symptoms of acute myocardial infarction are much less common in patients with diabetes. Consider cardiac ischaemia in a diabetic patient who describes shortness of breath (diastolic dysfunction), nausea/vomiting, sweating, even non-specific upper body discomfort. Patients are especially unlikely to use textbook terminology if English is not their first language.

Women in general, and especially older diabetic women, have worse outcomes because of a combination of more pronounced prior risk factors that remove pre-menopausal protection, atypical presenting symptoms, and delays throughout the ACS pathway.

Type 1 patients with a long duration of diabetes (e.g. >20 years) pose a particular challenge, because they may have no classical risk factors, and no evidence of advanced microvascular complications, unlike Type 2 patients, but can present at a relatively early age (in their 40s and 50s) with advanced calcific coronary artery disease, but again with only vague symptoms because of neuropathy.

ACS and heart failure are very common in patients with diabetic nephropathy and those on dialysis.

*The Hands-on Guide to Diabetes Care in Hospital*, First Edition by David Levy.
© 2016 John Wiley & Sons, Ltd. Published 2016 by John Wiley & Sons, Ltd.

## HEART FAILURE

Rapidly becoming the most common presentation of coronary artery disease in diabetes. Diabetic women are at about eightfold increased risk compared with non-diabetic women; diabetes is an independent risk factor for heart failure mortality. Emergency BNP or NT-pro BNP measurements, if available, are of value because of the wide differential in people with diabetes presenting with shortness of breath. However, around 30% of patients with heart failure and preserved ejection fraction (HFPEF) – especially common in Type 2 diabetes, and with a worse prognosis than heart failure with reduced ejection fraction – have normal biomarkers. Intensive glycaemic control has no impact on heart failure outcomes. 'Fatigue in the past few days' predicts hospital admission, but not mortality. Pulmonary embolism does not seem to be more common in diabetes, except in nephrotic and dialysis patients.

# 13 Acute coronary syndromes and stroke

**Top tip**

'Tight' glycaemic control (e.g. CBG 4–7 mmol/L) is of no short- or long-term benefit in acute cardiac cases. Target BG is the same as for all other acute medical patients – 7–10 mmol/L. There is nothing special about insulin in this situation.

**Key points**

*Acute coronary syndromes*

- Known diabetes (around 30%) and newly diagnosed diabetes (around 20%) are very common in patients presenting with ACS
- Try to make a diabetes diagnosis in all patients admitted with ACS; mortality is particularly high in people with previously undiagnosed diabetes. Admission BG >8 mmol/L adds significantly to the prognostic value of the GRACE score
- Neither tight glycaemic control nor routine intravenous insulin infusion (VRIII or GIK) improves outcomes in the acute phase of ACS
- Blood glucose target for ACS patients is the same as for all other acute medical patients, i.e. 7–10 mmol/L
- Any agents can be used to achieve this control – including metformin – but newly diagnosed patients with high blood glucose levels (e.g. persistently >11 mmol/L) should have insulin at least in the short-term
- Routine use of intravenous, followed by subcutaneous insulin, as in the DIGAMI study of 1997, is probably of no value in the modern era of ACS
- Female, insulin-requiring diabetic patients have an especially high in-hospital mortality rate but are more likely to be treated conservatively than getting the invasive treatment they will probably benefit from

*Stroke*

- Depending on the definition, up to 60% of ischaemic stroke patients will be hyperglycaemic
- Hyperglycaemia is associated with a worse clinical outcome and higher death rate than normoglycaemia
- Although there are some data that hyperglycaemic patients are at greater risk of symptomatic intracranial bleeding after thrombolysis, this is not confirmed in all studies, and hyperglycaemia or known diabetes should not prevent or delay thrombolysis if appropriate. Functional outcomes are much better in appropriately thrombolysed patients
- There is no evidence that in stroke patients reducing BG levels below the universal target (7–10 mmol/L) is of value; clinical trials continue

*The Hands-on Guide to Diabetes Care in Hospital,* First Edition by David Levy.
© 2016 John Wiley & Sons, Ltd. Published 2016 by John Wiley & Sons, Ltd.

## ACS

### Glycaemic diagnosis

Get a routine CBG measurement in all patients with suspected ACS and request an HbA$_{1c}$ early on in the admission. Around 20% will have undiagnosed diabetes (random CBG >11.1 or HbA$_{1c}$ ≥6.5% – **Chapter 3**), and 30% known diabetes, many in poor control. Some will have 'stress diabetes' (FBG >7.0 mmol/L or random BG >11.1 mmol/L, BUT HbA$_{1c}$ <6.5%). The prognosis in patients with previously undiagnosed diabetes is especially poor, probably because other vascular risk factors had gone undetected as well.

### The value of tight glycaemic control and insulin treatment

Neither 'tight' glycaemic control (target BG ~4–7 mmol/L) nor intravenous insulin in the acute phase confers any early or late cardiac benefit, and there are recurrent signals of harm in trials aiming for tight control. The DIGAMI study (1997), often quoted as showing the value of immediate i.v. insulin followed by 3 months of s.c. insulin, is now very old, and the nature of ACS and its treatment (immediate/early intervention compared with thrombolysis) have changed beyond recognition; the results are not transferable to the modern era of ACS management.

However, hyperglycaemia is a cardiovascular risk factor, and acute cardiac patients should have the same target for BG control as all other acute patients, i.e. 7–10 mmol/L. Try to achieve this quickly and maintain it – but avoid hypoglycaemia particularly assiduously in this situation. Hypoglycaemia is unpleasant and there is still a lingering concern about its potential to cause arrhythmias (speculative, but possibly associated with the 'dead in bed' syndrome in Type 1 diabetes, **Chapter 25**).

## PRACTICALITIES OF BLOOD GLUCOSE CONTROL IN ACS PATIENTS (Figure 13.1)

### Blood glucose testing

If eating, 7-point BG testing (fasting, before meals and 1½–2 hours after meals). All other patients should be tested at least 4-hourly.

### Known diabetes

- If eating: if BG levels are modestly elevated (e.g. up to 11 mmol/L), rapidly intensify existing treatment. If substantially elevated, e.g. consistently >12 mmol/L, start basal-bolus s.c. insulin. If uncontrolled, e.g. consistently >15 mmol/L, consider temporary VRIII with i.v. glucose.
- If not eating and BG >11 mmol/L, start VRIII.

### Newly diagnosed hyperglycaemia (either diabetes or 'stress hyperglycaemia')

Early in the admission it will not be clear whether this is 'stress hyperglycaemia' or newly-uncovered diabetes (the distinction will be evident once you get the HbA$_{1c}$). Remember the poor prognosis of these patients; patients with known diabetes do as well as non-diabetic people.

Start insulin if CBG consistently >12 mmol/L. This is not 'DIGAMI protocol'; it's trying to ensure reasonable glycaemic control in an acutely unwell diabetic person. Use an improvised basal-bolus regimen if the patient is eating (see **Chapter 22**). If not eating, use VRIII, but several studies have implicated high volumes of intravenous glucose in fluid overload, heart failure and hypokalaemia – resulting in poor acute outcomes. Start

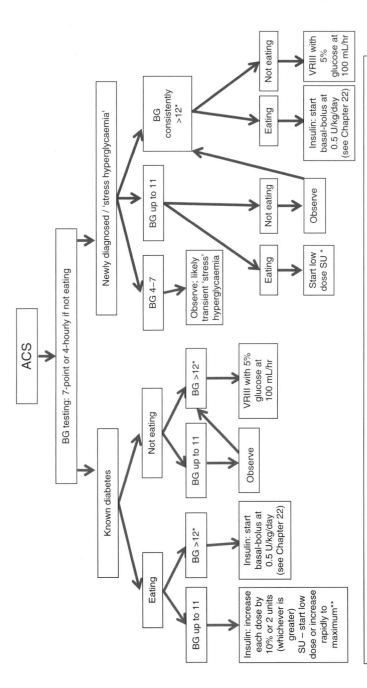

**Figure 13.1** Outline of glycaemic control in ACS patients.

*Cut points – the hazard of flow charts. Use these numbers with some flexibility, as there are no evidence-based thresholds for intervention.

** Gliclazide: start at 40 mg bd (once daily in the very thin or if unlikely to eat normally throughout the day). Maximum effective dose 240 mg daily. Leave metformin, if taken, at the admission dose, unless there are indications to discontinue it. Do not increase the dose, as it acts too slowly in this acute situation.

with 100 mL 5% glucose hourly, discontinue as soon as possible, check creatinine and electrolytes daily, and ensure [K$^+$] 3.5–4.5 mmol/L.

Allow BG levels up to 11 mmol/L without starting treatment – treating BG lower than this in patients with an unclear diagnosis risks hypoglycaemia, especially if this is transient 'stress'-type hyperglycaemia.

### Diabetic patients treated with non-insulin agents (see Chapter 24)
Other treatments can remain unchanged, but note:

- Metformin: modify dose if renal function has deteriorated, and discontinue if eGFR <30 mL/min. Discontinue for 48 hours after angiography and reinstate so long as serum creatinine has not risen by >25%. There is a widespread mistaken view that metformin is itself nephrotoxic, and some patients are told this. Educate patients and other HCPs on this example of diabetes mythology
- Discontinue pioglitazone because of the risk of fluid retention

Establishing a permanent diabetes medication regime in these patients is difficult. Many will have arrived in hospital on little or no medication, but will go home with a very long prescription list. Simplicity is critical and if BG levels are <11 mmol/L, try to avoid insulin (this is a point on which the evidence base and patient preference are almost perfectly congruent). Remember that insulin confers no specific cardiac advantage; don't allow cardiologists to tell you otherwise.

## REVASCULARISATION STRATEGIES IN DIABETIC ACS PATIENTS
You will not be managing STEMI patients unless you work at a cardiac centre. NSTEMI patients with diabetes are less likely to have a recurrent nonfatal MI than non-diabetic patients if they receive an invasive strategy (with an absolute likelihood of a better outcome), but they are less likely to receive such treatment, especially if female and insulin-treated.

### Multi-vessel disease and CABG
Diabetic patients with known multi-vessel disease (whether or not insulin treated) and not offered invasive treatment during their index admission will benefit from CABG (lower mortality and MI risk at 3 years). Stenting is associated with a high rate of re-intervention and major cardiac and cerebral vascular events at 3–5 years.

While you will not be making these clinical decisions yourself, you are an advocate for your patients, and you should discuss the clinical situation with the cardiologists. They should be gently and politely asked the evidence base supporting their decision.

## STROKE

Don't withhold thrombolysis from a hyperglycaemic patient. There is no conclusive evidence of harm, and functional benefits are probably as great as in non-diabetic patients

Through various pathways, hyperglycaemia is a risk factor for increased severity of brain infarction, and worse outcomes for functional improvement and mortality. As with ACS, impaired glucose tolerance is found in about 40% of stroke patients, and diabetes in about 20%, but transient hyperglycaemia after acute stroke is very common too, usually settling within 8 hours.

## Thrombolysis

There is concern about an increased risk of symptomatic post-thrombolysis intracerebral haemorrhage in diabetic patients; reperfusion injury may be more common in hyperglycaemia. However, functional improvement after thrombolysis is similar in all patients, and the consensus is that thrombolysis should not be withheld in hyperglycaemic patients.

## Acute glucose control during stroke

Trials of tight control have either shown no benefit or have not recruited sufficient patients. Until there is more definitive guidance, target the same BG level as in any other hospitalised patient (i.e. 7–10 mmol/L), but there is a case for slightly more lax control, especially in patients who have diminished conscious levels (or fits). If you plan VRIII for a severely hyperglycaemic patient (e.g. BG consistently >15 mmol/L), ensure they are admitted to a sufficiently high dependency area where hourly BG monitoring can be guaranteed. Review the VRIII scale frequently to avoid any hint of hypoglycaemia.

### Further reading

Goyal A, Spertus JA, Gosch K, et al. Serum potassium levels and mortality in acute myocardial infarction. *JAMA* 2012;307:157–64. PMID: 22235085.

Malmberg K. Prospective randomised study of intensive insulin treatment on long term survival after acute myocardial infarction in patients with diabetes mellitus. DIGAMI (Diabetes Mellitus, Insulin Glucose Infusion in Acute Myocardial Infarction) Study Group. *BMJ*. 1997;314:1512-5. PMID: 9169397.

O'Donoghue ML, Vaidya A, Afsal R, et al. An invasive or conservative in patients with diabetes mellitus and non-ST-segment elevation acute coronary syndromes: a collaborative meta-analysis of randomized trials. *J Am Coll Cardiol*. 2012;60:106–11. PMID: 22766336.

# 14 Secondary prevention after ACS

**Top tip**

Glycaemic control is probably less important than LDL cholesterol and BP control in the post-ACS patient, but always aim for HbA$_{1c}$ <8.0% (64 mmol/mol). Do everything you can to avoid hypoglycaemia.

**Key points**

- People with diabetes are at high risk of second and subsequent coronary events
- Discuss with your patients the importance of obsessive attention to secondary prevention measures
- Medical risk factors in order of importance: lipid-lowering, BP control, antiplatelet treatment, glycaemic control
- Other medication: angiotensin blockade, beta blockade
- Lifestyle adjustments in order of importance: smoking cessation, exercise and diet

## TABLE OF CHECKLIST ITEMS (Table 14.1)

**Table 14.1** Important elements of secondary coronary prevention

| Lifestyle | Medication | Comments |
|---|---|---|
| • Cardiac rehabilitation and exercise training <br> • Smoking cessation (whole family) <br> • Diet portfolio (weight loss and specific dietary items) | • Glycaemia <br><br> • BP <br><br> • Lipids – statins <br> • Angiotensin blockade (ACE-i or ARB) <br> • Antiplatelet treatment <br> • Beta-blocker | • HbA$_{1c}$ <8%. No specific benefit of insulin <br> • <140/80 (casual) <br><br> • Intensive statin treatment e.g. atorvastatin 40 or 80 mg daily, target LDL <1.7–1.8 mmol/L, lower probably better |

The importance of implementing a comprehensive package of secondary prevention measures – medication and lifestyle – cannot be overstated, and is crucial in reducing the very high risk of recurrent events in people with diabetes (relative risk at least 1.5 compared with non-diabetic patients). Pressured hospital staff are more enthusiastic about medication than discussing lifestyle, but brief education in the immediate post-MI period

*The Hands-on Guide to Diabetes Care in Hospital,* First Edition by David Levy.
© 2016 John Wiley & Sons, Ltd. Published 2016 by John Wiley & Sons, Ltd.

is probably effective in improving long-term adherence (for example, in smoking cessation). Most studies depressingly confirm that many patients stop taking their medication surprisingly quickly after the index event, and adherence with all preventative treatments falls to about 50% after a year.

### Lifestyle adjustments

Much of the advice will be given by other members of the cardiac team, but patients will likely ask your opinion. It's best if you have some kind of evidence base for your advice.

**Exercise: cardiac rehabilitation and exercise training:**  Ensure you know your hospital's local arrangements. Home delivery of rehabilitation post-myocardial infarction is as effective as and more economical than at a formal centre, but training and reinforcement are critical.

**Smoking cessation:**  If your hospital has a smoking cessation service, use it fully (and take the opportunity to counsel smoking members of the patients' families, not forgetting the risks of passive smoking). Patients receiving counselling gain a significant mortality benefit. Weirdly, diabetic patients seem *less* likely to receive inpatient counselling. Target them specifically: successfully managing any risk factor will carry particular benefits in diabetic patients because of their higher absolute risk.

**Diet:**  There is limited RCT evidence, but adherence to a portfolio of diet advice and weight control is likely to be useful:

- Weight reduction: target BMI <25, or 10% weight loss (very difficult) if initial BMI is >27.5. High dose insulin in Type 2 diabetes makes weight loss more difficult. Judicious juggling with non-insulin medications can help, as can targeted reductions in insulin doses. Ask for diabetes team advice if the patient is taking insulin at a higher dose than 1 U/kg/day
- The traditional 'Mediterranean' diet has cardiovascular (and cancer-reducing) benefits (olive oil, vegetables, fish, low animal protein, low fat dairy produce)
- Low total and saturated fat (there is no convincing evidence for this, and it is not included in current USA guidelines)
- Low salt
- Recommended alcohol intake where appropriate and acceptable
- Increase soluble and insoluble fibre
- Increased oily fish (at least 2 portions per week); in recent studies, fish oil supplements (over the counter or prescribable) are of no value
- Avoid 'antioxidant' vitamin supplements
- ?50 g dark (≥70% cocoa) chocolate per day

### Medication

**Lipids:**  Numerical LDL targets (e.g. <1.7–1.8 mmol/L) are under evidence-based fire from advocates of intensity of lipid lowering (moderate: simvastatin/pravastatin *vs* intensive: atorvastatin/rosuvastatin). This is the approach used in acute care, where intensive statin treatment started in hospital or shortly after reduces fatal and recurrent events. Compliance is higher if statin treatment starts in hospital. High dose atorvastatin (40 or 80 mg daily) has a good safety record in this situation. Mention to patients sceptical of the benefits of statins that 5 years of treatment reduce events and possibly mortality up to 20 years later.

Muscle side-effects are more frequent with simvastatin and atorvastatin than with pravastatin and rosuvastatin. Do not change from simvastatin to atorvastatin if a patient has had previous side-effects with simvastatin – where available start rosuvastatin 20 mg daily.

*Other lipid-modifying drugs*    All attempts to reduce the high residual cardiovascular risk in diabetic patients by drug treatment of the diabetic dyslipidaemia – high triglycerides (>1.7 mmol/L) and low HDL-cholesterol (<1.0 mmol/L in men, <1.3 in women) – have been unsuccessful. Several RCTs confirm that broadly speaking only statins and ezetimibe confer prognostic benefit, though other agents may 'improve' the numbers. These include fibric acid drugs (bezafibrate, fenofibrate), niacin and omega-3 fatty acids (fish oils) – unless triglycerides are so high (possibly >5 mmol/L, definitely >10 mmol/L) that there is a pancreatitis risk, where a fibrate should be started (e.g. m/r bezafibrate 400 mg daily).

## Angiotensin blockade
Routine full-dose angiotensin blockade is recommended, its cardioprotective effects probably greater than can be accounted for by their usually minor antihypertensive effects (especially in patients with low baseline blood pressure). Treatment is mandatory in patients with any degree of heart failure. Cardioprotection is probably better with ACE-inhibitor treatment than angiotensin receptor blockade.

### Starting doses
- ACE-inhibitors: ramipril 2.5 mg daily, lisinopril 5 mg daily, perindopril 4 mg daily.
- ARBs: losartan 50 mg daily, irbesartan 150 mg daily, valsartan 80 mg daily.

ARBs are more prone than ACE-inhibitors to cause postural hypotension.

The risks of dual angiotensin blockade (ACE-inhibitor + ARB) for any indication (hypertension, heart failure, diabetic nephropathy) far outweigh the benefits. Discontinue the ARB in patients taking dual blockade and maximise the dose of ACE-inhibitor, if necessary.

## Antiplatelet agents
Low dose aspirin for primary prevention in Type 2 patients is no longer recommended, but few of your patients will fall into this category. The protocols in secondary prevention are complex, but they are summarised in **Table 14.2**.

**Table 14.2** Antiplatelet regimens in patients with CAD (Dr Francesco Papalia, Barts Heart Centre)

| Coronary intervention | Aspirin | Diabetes | | Non-diabetes | |
|---|---|---|---|---|---|
| | | P2Y12 inhibitor? | Duration | P2Y12 inhibitor? | Duration |
| STEMI no PCI | Lifelong for all patients | Yes (clopidogrel/ ticagrelor only) | 4 weeks | Yes (clopidogrel/ ticagrelor only) | 4 weeks |
| STEMI + DES | | Yes (?prasugrel first line) | 12 months | Yes | 12 months |
| STEMI + BMS | | Yes (?prasugrel first line) | 4 weeks | Yes | 4 weeks |
| NSTEACS no PCI | | Yes (clopidogrel/ ticagrelor only) | 12 months | Yes (clopidogrel/ ticagrelor only) | 12 months |
| NSTEACS + DES | | Yes (?prasugrel first line) | 12 months | Yes | 12 months |
| NSTEACS + BMS | | Yes (?prasugrel first line) | 12 months | Yes | 12 months |
| Stable CAD | No | – | | No | – |
| Post-CABG | No | – | | No | – |

## Beta-blockers

Of unequivocal value in patients with poor LV function, but their value is less clear in lower risk patients, in whom a year of treatment is probably sufficient. The doses in current use are a pallid reflection of those used in clinical trials (e.g. metoprolol 100 mg bd). Diabetes hasn't been a contraindication to beta blockers for decades. They do not cause or further impair hypoglycaemia unawareness (a myth that refuses to lie down), do not exacerbate peripheral vascular disease (another one — other than cause cold feet when used in high doses), and although large-scale studies show they may slightly raise glucose levels and impair lipid profiles, these are of no concern in the individual patient, nor should they be to the individual physician.

### Further reading

Boden WE, O'Rourke RA, Teo KK, et al.; COURAGE Trial Research Group. Optimal medical therapy with or without PCI for stable coronary disease. *N Engl J Med.* 2007;356:1503–16. PMID: 17387127.

# 15 Acute pancreatitis

**Key points**

- Type 2 diabetes carries increased risks of acute pancreatitis (AP), though the risk seems to be lower in insulin-treated patients (**Figure 15.1**)
- 10% of AP is associated with hypertriglyceridaemia, which itself may be secondary to newly diagnosed or established and poorly controlled diabetes
- Gallstones and alcohol are – as in non-diabetic patients – the commonest causes of AP. Alcohol is frequently itself associated with high triglyceride levels
- Even though most cases of triglyceride-induced pancreatitis do not occur in people with diabetes, hyperglycaemia – because of transient or permanent β-cell destruction – is common in all patients with pancreatitis
- Therefore – most cases of acute pancreatitis should be treated with VRIII, with or without high-concentration glucose; intensive insulin treatment may reduce length of stay
- In severely hypertriglyceridaemic states, consider treatment with intravenous unfractionated heparin at ~500 U/hr. Insulin and heparin both suppress hypertriglyceridaemia
- Pancreatitis is still managed as a 'surgical' emergency, although urgent surgery is almost never needed. Because patients are admitted to surgical wards, the necessary medical input can be intermittent. Be aware of this, and ensure that the diabetes team is always informed about AP cases

## HYPERGLYCAEMIA DURING AND AFTER AP

Type 2 diabetes doubles the risk of developing AP, but most patients are admitted without a prior diagnosis of diabetes. Routinely monitor all AP patients with 4-hourly BG and an admission $HbA_{1c}$. Transient hyperglycaemia during admission is very common and does not always settle after discharge. About 15% of patients develop diabetes within 12 months, many requiring insulin treatment. Five years after the acute episode, diabetes risk increases nearly threefold. Make a plan for diabetes surveillance in patients who had new-onset hyperglycaemia during AP – for example, request their GP to do an $HbA_{1c}$ every 4 months.

## ABDOMINAL PAIN AND HYPERGLYCAEMIA

Patients with upper abdominal pain and elevated blood glucose levels (>11 mmol/L) pose a problem of differential diagnosis:

**Diabetic ketoacidosis** – venous blood gases, serum amylase and urinary or preferably capillary blood ketones. Recall that new Type 1 diabetes can occur in middle-aged or non-white patients. Elevated amylase in DKA (e.g. up to 3 × upper limit of laboratory reference value), and abdominal pain is associated with low pH and high osmolarity. Ask for a surgical review, but in most cases, symptoms settle with the metabolic state.

*The Hands-on Guide to Diabetes Care in Hospital,* First Edition by David Levy.
© 2016 John Wiley & Sons, Ltd. Published 2016 by John Wiley & Sons, Ltd.

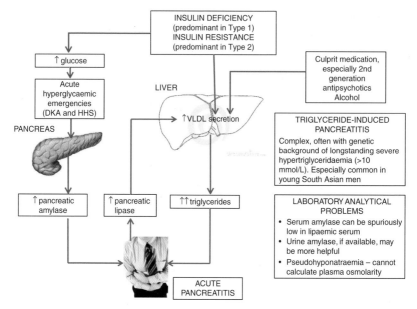

**Figure 15.1** The clinical and pathological relationships between diabetes, elevated triglycerides and acute pancreatitis.

**Triglyceride-induced pancreatitis** carries the same prognosis as pancreatitis from any other cause (it may be worse because of the proliferation of metabolic abnormalities and there is a high risk of recurrence). If blood is lipaemic on venesection, then treat amylase levels in all patients with suspicion, and get an abdominal CT scan (looking for bulky pancreas, fat stranding; gall stones: **Figures 15.2** and **15.3**).

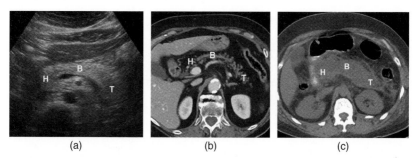

(a)                                    (b)                                    (c)

**Figure 15.2** CT scan is the first-line radiological investigation for suspected acute pancreatitis. (a) Contrast enhanced axial CT image of normal pancreas (head [H], body [B], tail [T]). (b) Compare (a) with the chronic atrophic pancreatitis often seen in long-standing Type 1 diabetes, though exocrine insufficiency in uncomplicated Type 1 diabetes almost never occurs. (c) Nonenhanced axial CT image showing a swollen pancreas, and inflammatory changes in the peri-pancreatic fat. *Source*: Reproduced with permission of Sergei Kuzmich, Whipps Cross University Hospital.

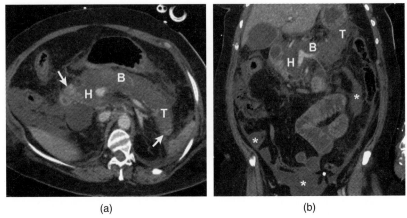

(a)                                           (b)

**Figure 15.3** Severe necrotizing pancreatitis. (a) Contrast enhanced axial CT image showing severe pancreatic necrosis – there is almost no enhancement in the pancreas, except for small areas of the head and tail (arrows). (b) Contrast enhanced coronal CT image showing collections of fluid around the abdomen (asterisks) in addition to the pancreatic necrosis. *Source*: Reproduced with permission of Sergei Kuzmich, Whipps Cross University Hospital.

### Other factors:

- Alcohol – the commonest cause of acute pancreatitis
- Drugs, many of which have been anecdotally implicated in acute pancreatitis. Be especially vigilant in patients who are at risk of the metabolic syndrome (obesity, ethnic minority, family history of diabetes) and also taking antipsychotic medication (notably olanzapine, clozapine, risperidone and possibly quetiapine, though the conventional agents seem to pose a greater risk)
- Thiazides, glucocorticoids and the oral contraceptive, while commonly cited as causes are rarely implicated in practice
- There has been much discussion over the risk of acute pancreatitis with the use of the incretin-related antidiabetes agents – DPP4 inhibitors (gliptins) and GLP-1 analogues (see **Chapter 24**). If there is any risk, it is small
- Ensure that any of these agents are discontinued in patients with AP, and not reinstated

## MANAGEMENT OF DIABETES

### During admission

Four-hourly CBG and admission $HbA_{1c}$ are needed in all patients with AP.

Many patients will require enteral nutrition (starting it within 48 hours may be of long-term benefit). Insulin is mandatory here (see **Chapter 28**), and often in high doses because of the acquired insulin resistance of the illness, together with the high glycaemic load of enteral feeds. VRIII or high-dose subcutaneous insulin are both appropriate. If using subcutaneous insulin start no lower than 0.5 U/kg/day, divided according to the feeding regime, and plan to increase daily in response to post-feed capillary glucose levels.

### At discharge

Always bear in mind the possibility of exocrine insufficiency (symptoms of malabsorption, progressive weight loss); this is another reason for careful follow-up after an episode of AP.

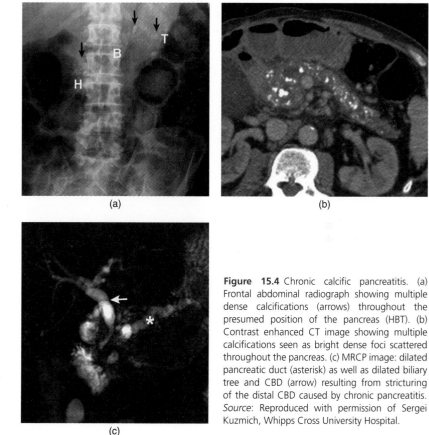

**Figure 15.4** Chronic calcific pancreatitis. (a) Frontal abdominal radiograph showing multiple dense calcifications (arrows) throughout the presumed position of the pancreas (HBT). (b) Contrast enhanced CT image showing multiple calcifications seen as bright dense foci scattered throughout the pancreas. (c) MRCP image: dilated pancreatic duct (asterisk) as well as dilated biliary tree and CBD (arrow) resulting from stricturing of the distal CBD caused by chronic pancreatitis. *Source*: Reproduced with permission of Sergei Kuzmich, Whipps Cross University Hospital.

## Chronic calcific pancreatitis with malabsorption (Figure 15.4)

This appears to be getting more common in people with longstanding Type 2 diabetes. Although there is little literature, look out for it in thin, insulin-requiring Type 2 patients with malabsorptive symptoms, and also in patients with increasing hypoglycaemia frequency and decreasing insulin requirements. Coeliac disease would be uncommon in this group, but always exclude Addison's disease with a short synacthen test.

### Pancreatic diabetes and insulin treatment

Pancreatic diabetes can be very taxing for everyone. Patients can be of Type 2 phenotype and insulin resistant, while at the same time have marked insulin deficiency as a result of chronic pancreatic disease. Because they are often deficient in glucagon as well as insulin – unlike autoimmune Type 1 diabetes – they lack the primary defence against hypoglycaemia. Unfortunately, poor overall glycaemic control associated with high risk of hypoglycaemia is the result in many patients. The micro- and macrovascular complications of pancreatic diabetes are as severe as in other forms of diabetes. If there is associated alcoholism, chronic cigarette smoking or long-term psychiatric illness, management becomes a major challenge.

# 16 Infections in diabetes

**Key points**

- Diabetes is associated with increased infection risk and an array of uncommon infections
- Common infections (soft tissue, bone, urinary tract and chest) respond less predictably than in people without diabetes
- Extended durations of antimicrobial treatment are often warranted
- Liaise with your microbiology colleagues, but hospital antimicrobial guidelines do not always emphasise the specific risks of infections in diabetes
- Don't underestimate the risk of progression and complications of infection (especially soft tissue and visceral), and if in doubt admit the patient to confirm the diagnosis and plan management
- Infected foot ulcers can only be treated in the community if there is a watertight antimicrobial schedule that does not compromise efficacy for expediency
- Ensure all diabetic patients are up to date on their immunisations and that they understand their importance

Diabetes probably increases the risks of most infections. The risks are massively increased in dialysis patients, especially infections that are unusual in non-diabetic people, for example, acute endocarditis caused by *Staphylococcus aureus*, and splenic abscesses (sometimes together). Tuberculosis and diabetes were closely linked in the early days of insulin treatment, and the association now seems to be re-emerging.

## SOFT TISSUE INFECTIONS

### Cellulitis
- Commonest organisms: *S. aureus*, β-haemolytic streptococci, usually group A
- Cellulitis is more common, involves more tissue and is more resistant to treatment in people with diabetes. Gas-forming organisms are obviously serious
- Always examine the leg carefully: 'red leg' with no infection is common after repeated episodes of cellulitis

*The Hands-on Guide to Diabetes Care in Hospital,* First Edition by David Levy.
© 2016 John Wiley & Sons, Ltd. Published 2016 by John Wiley & Sons, Ltd.

- Most patients need intravenous antibiotics either as an inpatient or in the community (hospital at home, or similar if available). Readmission following failure to resolve on with oral antibiotics is common
- Infections not involving the leg can be treated with oral antibiotics. Admit all patients with cellulitis associated with foot ulcers
- Peripheral oedema inhibits resolution of infection: loop diuretics and bed rest/elevating the leg are important
- Blood cultures are usually negative. Culture fluid from unruptured blisters

## TREATMENT (Table 16.1)

### Oral antibiotics – 7 days

- Co-amoxiclav 625 tds or ciprofloxacin 500 mg bd (where permitted)
- Clindamycin 300–450 mg qds in penicillin-sensitive
- Oral macrolides (erythromycin, clarithromycin) are probably not potent enough
- Metronidazole is not necessary (if you suspect an anaerobic infection, there is an abscess, and the patient needs surgery)

### Intravenous antibiotics – 5–7 days

- Benzylpenicillin and flucloxacillin 1 g each qds
- Co-amoxiclav 1.2 g tds
- Clindamycin 300–450 mg qds in penicillin-sensitive
- Vancomycin 1 g bd in MRSA or suspected MRSA, or penicillin-sensitive

Systemically unwell patients who have had previous antibiotic treatment: ceftazidime (1–2 g tds) until more specific advice and culture results are available.
Patients often require 2–4 weeks of intravenous treatment if there is a large amount of infected tissue. If there is no or little response to benzylpenicillin/flucloxacillin after 3–4 days, add high-dose clindamycin.

## NECROTIZING FASCIITIS

Fulminating gangrene of the skin caused by rapidly spreading microvascular thrombosis affecting subcutaneous fat, dermis and muscle. Thirty per cent of cases have associated diabetes. It usually occurs in the limbs, but feet, face and neck (often of dental origin) can be involved (**Figure 16.1**). Fournier's gangrene is a specific form involving the perineum, genitalia and perianal area (**Figure 16.2**), and it is also described in the neck (again dental origin). Organism is usually Lancefield group A β-haemolytic streptococcus.
At onset, the signs may be little different from cellulitis, but irregular dusky blue and black patches appear and extend rapidly.
Point of care ultrasound may be helpful (**Figure 16.1a**); CT is diagnostic. Get an immediate surgical and ICU opinion; without surgery, multiorgan failure and death are inevitable.

### Warning features of necrotising fasciitis

- Any extensive pre-existing area of infection in a diabetic leg or foot, e.g. heel ulcer, wet gangrene with spreading cellulitis
- Fever
- Laboratory findings: rising white count, rising creatinine, elevated potassium secondary to cell necrosis
- Patients need urgent surgery: this situation can't wait until the next day

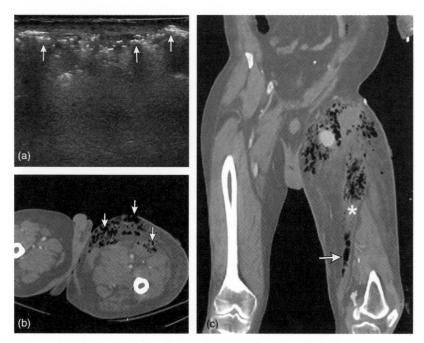

**Figure 16.1** Necrotising fasciitis. (a) Ultrasound image of the left groin showing multiple pockets of soft tissue gas (arrows). This establishes the diagnosis as a major emergency, but CT is needed to show extent. (b) Corresponding axial CT confirming multiple soft tissue gas pockets. (c) Coronal reformatted CT image of left thigh. Gas pockets are tracking from the groin to the upper knee. There is gas in the sartorius muscle (asterisk) that extends into its insertion (arrow). *Source*: Reproduced with permission of Sergei Kuzmich, Whipps Cross University Hospital.

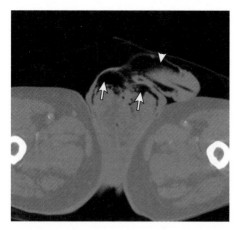

**Figure 16.2** Fournier gangrene. Unenhanced axial CT image showing multiple widespread pockets of gas in the soft tissues of the scrotum (arrows) and penis (arrowhead) originating from perineal sepsis. *Source*: Reproduced with permission of Sergei Kuzmich, Whipps Cross University Hospital.

**Table 16.1** Summary of antibiotic treatment for soft tissue infections in diabetes with dosage adjustments in renal impairment: initially use only intravenous agents in ulcer patients

| | | Relative activity against specific pathogens | | | | | | Dosage adjustments in renal impairment | |
| | Starting dose | S aureus | Strep | Entero | Anaer | Comments | | eGFR or GFR (mL/min) | Dose |
|---|---|---|---|---|---|---|---|---|---|
| **Oral antibiotic*** | | | | | | | | | |
| Co-amoxiclav | 625 mg tds | ++++ | ++++ | ++ | +++ | Important broad-spectrum antibiotic | | | As in normal renal function |
| Ciprofloxacin | 500 mg bd | +++ | ++ | ++++ | 0 | Good bone penetration in osteomyelitis risk; generally well-tolerated but ↑Clostridium difficile risk | | 30–60<br><30 | 250–500 mg 12 hourly<br>250–500 mg 24  hourly |
| Levofloxacin | 500 mg od or bd | +++ | ++ | ++++ | + | | | 20–50<br><br><20 | Initial dose 250–500 mg, then 125 mg 12–24 hourly<br>Initial dose 250–500 mg, then 125 mg 12–48 hourly |
| Clindamycin | 300–450 mg qds | ++++ | +++ | 0 | ++++ | Good bone penetration. Important anti-staphylococcal agent. Possible ↑C. diff risk, but approved because of narrow spectrum | | | As in normal renal function |
| Metronidazole | 400 mg tds | 0 | 0 | 0 | ++++ | Anti-anaerobic only. Use in abscesses and ischaemic lesions, but not as a routine | | | As in normal renal function |
| **Intravenous antibiotic** | | | | | | | | | |
| Co-amoxiclav | 1.2 g qds | ++++ | ++++ | ++ | +++ | Probably best first-line treatment, especially in patients who have had recent oral antibiotic(s) | | 10–30<br><10 | 1.2 g 12 hourly<br>1.2 g initially, then 600 mg 8 hourly or 1.2 g 12 hourly |

*(Continued)*

**Table 16.1** (Continued)

| | Starting dose | Relative activity against specific pathogens | | | | Comments | Dosage adjustments in renal impairment | |
| | | S aureus | Strep | Entero | Anaer | | eGFR or GFR (mL/ min) | Dose |
| --- | --- | --- | --- | --- | --- | --- | --- | --- |
| Benzylpenicillin | 1.2 g qds | + | ++++ | + | ++ | With flucloxacillin, the usual recommended initial combination, but it is cumbersome and time-consuming for nursing staff | 20–50 <br> <10–20 | As in normal renal function <br> 600 mg–1.2 g 6 hourly depending on severity of infection |
| Flucloxacillin | 1 g qds | ++++ | ++++ | 0 | ++ | As benzylpenicillin; watch liver function in long-term use | | Up to 4 g daily, as in normal renal function |
| Piperacillin/ tazobactam | 4.5 g tds | ++++ | ++++ | +++ | ++++ | Very broad spectrum, including Pseudomonas spp. | <20 | 4.5 g 12 hourly |
| Imipenem/ cilastatin | 500 mg qds or 1 g tds, max 1 g qds | ++++ | ++++ | ++++ | +++ | As piperacillin/tazobactam | 41–70 <br> 21–40 <br> <20 | 500 mg 6–8 hourly or 750 mg 8 hourly <br> 250 mg 6 hourly or 500 mg 6–8 hourly <br> 250–500 mg (or 4.5 mg/kg, whichever is lower) 12 hourly |
| Ciprofloxacin | 400 mg bd | +++ | ++ | ++++ | 0 | As for oral preparation | 30–60 <br> <30 | 200–400 mg 12 hourly <br> 200–400 mg 24 hourly |
| Levofloxacin | 500 mg od or bd | +++ | +++ | ++++ | + | As for oral preparation | 20–50 <br> <20 | 250–500 mg initially, then 125 mg 12–24 hourly <br> 250–500 mg initially, then 125 mg 12–48 hourly |
| Cefuroxime | 750 mg tds | ++++ | ++++ | ++ | ++ | Less approved (C. diff) | 10–20 <br> <10 | 750 mg 12 hourly <br> 750 mg 24 hourly |
| Ceftriaxone | 1 g daily, 2–4 g daily in severe infections | +++ | +++ | ++++ | ++ | Valuable in severe infections in penicillin-sensitive patients, or when mixed organisms are suspected (e.g. multiple recent courses of antibiotics) | <10 | Maximum 2 g daily |

(Continued)

| | Starting dose | Relative activity against specific pathogens | | | | | Dosage adjustments in renal impairment | |
| | | S aureus | Strep | Entero | Anaer | Comments | eGFR or GFR (mL/min) | Dose |
|---|---|---|---|---|---|---|---|---|
| Ceftazidime | 1–2 g tds | +++ | +++ | ++++ | ++ | | 31–50<br>16–30<br>6–15<br><5 | 1–2 g 12 hourly<br>1–2 g 24 hourly<br>500 mg – 1 g 24 hourly<br>500 mg – 1 g 48 hourly |
| Clindamycin | 300–900 mg tds | ++++ | +++ | 0 | ++++ | Valuable monotherapy in penicillin-sensitive patients with uncomplicated cellulitis; similar spectrum to vancomycin | | As in normal renal function |
| Metronidazole | 500 mg tds | 0 | 0 | 0 | ++++ | As for oral preparation | | |
| Vancomycin | 1 g bd ( >65 years, 500 mg bd or 1 g od) | ++++ | +++ | 0 | ++ | MRSA or penicillin-sensitive patients | 20–50<br>10–20<br><10 | 500 mg – 1 g 12–24 hourly<br>500 mg – 1 g 24–48 hourly<br>500 mg – 1 g 48–96 hourly<br>Monitor pre-dose (trough) level, which should be 10–15 mg/L |

*Phenoxymethylpenicillin (penicillin V) and the macrolides (erythromycin, clarithromycin) are not potent enough for use in this situation.

Strep = Streptococci; Entero = enterobacteriaceae (e.g. *Enterobacter, E. coli, Morganella, Proteus, Salmonella, Serratia*); Anaer = anaerobes.

Dosages in renal impairment are taken either from the BNF or The Renal Drug Handbook, 4th edition – whichever gives the simpler information. The Renal Drug Handbook quotes renal function as GFR (creatinine clearance), but for practical purposes, eGFR and GFR are here used interchangeably.

*Source:* Reproduced with permission of Ching Yee Ngan, Medicines Optimisation Pharmacist, Barts Health NHS Trust.

## DIABETIC FOOT ULCERS

- Examine the feet (**Figure 16.3**) and record your findings on a simple diagram. In order to do this reliably, it is nearly always best to remove the patient's shoes and socks and any wound dressings.
- Diagnose the problem:
  - 75% of ulcers are neuropathic
  - Punched-out plantar ulcers overlying the 1st or 4th/5th metatarsal head pressure areas are always neuropathic
  - Toe and heel ulcers and ulcers on the dorsum of the foot or lateral or medial sides of the feet are usually ischaemic, and are often caused by acute trauma, for example, newly acquired badly fitting shoes
  - 'Sausage toe' – swollen, dusky/ischaemic digit resulting from local sepsis-related thrombosis usually means underlying osteomyelitis – look carefully for radiological signs, which may be difficult to spot in the phalanges. Large-vessel ischaemia may be present, but is not the immediate cause

## ADMISSION

### In general, think twice before discharging a patient from ED

Because of neuropathy, and poor mobility and vision, patients present late. Sadly, but characteristically, the first symptoms may be odour or serosanguinous fluid in footwear or socks. If you're inclined to discharge the patient, consider the symptoms you might have with a 4-cm foot ulcer eroding to the bone.

### Always admit

- Patients with ischaemic lesions (dusky, blotchy, frankly gangrenous), regardless of size
- Dialysis patients (risk of rapid progression and systemic infection; usually numb neuro-pathic feet; sometimes severe visual impairment)
- Nearly all patients with an infected neuropathic ulcer

Patients with infected ulcers can be discharged if there is no more than 2 cm of cellulitis around the ulcer, but infections can proceed very rapidly, especially in unsupervised patients on their own at home. They are commonly seen by a different team and readmitted a few days after discharge with worsening infection because of inadequate antibiotic treatment and imprecise follow-up arrangements that never had any chance of working for the patient. Request CRP (<17 mg/L suggests there is no significant infection) and foot X-ray. You never know when or where osteomyelitis is lurking, and antibiotics alone are not sufficient – offloading and meticulous wound care are needed as well.

### Before discharge from ED

- Ensure there is a referral to either the community podiatry team (if the patient is already being supervised in the community) or the hospital team (if this is a first presentation). Do not refer back to general practice or to a general community nursing team.
- Remind the patient to come back if the infection worsens (remember these patients are usually neuropathic, so pain is not a reliable symptom). Someone needs to look at the foot for the patient.
- Write a prescription for antibiotics that can be immediately filled (co-amoxiclav 625 i tds for a week; ciprofloxacin 500 mg bd or clindamycin 300 mg tds in penicillin-sensitive).

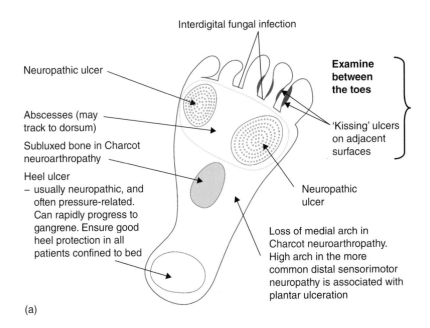

Interdigital fungal infection

Neuropathic ulcer

**Examine between the toes**

Abscesses (may track to dorsum)

Subluxed bone in Charcot neuroarthropathy

Heel ulcer
– usually neuropathic, and often pressure-related. Can rapidly progress to gangrene. Ensure good heel protection in all patients confined to bed

'Kissing' ulcers on adjacent surfaces

Neuropathic ulcer

Loss of medial arch in Charcot neuroarthropathy. High arch in the more common distal sensorimotor neuropathy is associated with plantar ulceration

(a)

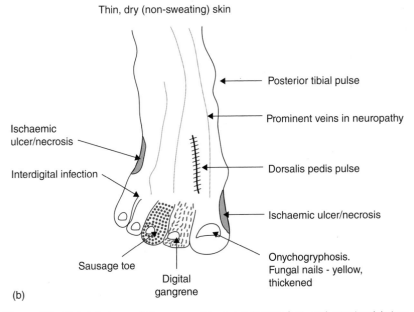

Thin, dry (non-sweating) skin

Posterior tibial pulse

Prominent veins in neuropathy

Ischaemic ulcer/necrosis

Interdigital infection

Dorsalis pedis pulse

Ischaemic ulcer/necrosis

Onychogryphosis. Fungal nails - yellow, thickened

Sausage toe

Digital gangrene

(b)

**Figure 16.3** Clinical features of the neuropathic and ischaemic foot, and associated lesions. (a) Plantar view. (b) Dorsal view. Remove all dressings. Document your findings, and in patients with extensive ulceration, request medical photography as soon as possible.

## If admitting

- Admit to a medical ward: if this is the first admission with an ulcer, you should tell the patient they are likely to be in hospital for at least 2 weeks.
- Get a foot X-ray – look for osteomyelitis, gas in the tissues, possible Charcot neuroarthropathy. Indicate the site of any ulcer on the request form – osteomyelitis usually occurs in bones adjacent to the ulcer, but early radiological signs are easily overlooked.
- Confirm doses of antibiotics, adjust for renal dysfunction. Write up antibiotics and ensure the first dose is given (**Table 16.1**).
- If there is clear evidence of ischaemia, submit a request for imaging: CT angiography, or unenhanced MRA in patients with acute kidney injury or eGFR <30 mL/min or on dialysis (risk of nephrogenic systemic fibrosis with gadolinium-based contrast media; no risk with CKD stages 1–3).

## Communications

Surgical responsibility for managing diabetic foot problems differs between hospitals (vascular surgeons or orthopaedic surgeons; commonly now admitting surgical team of the week). Unless there are orthopaedic surgeons with a special interest in the foot and ankle, the vascular surgeons and diabetes team are your best bet for first stop advice: surgery for abscesses and excluding remediable vascular lesions are priorities.

Inform the diabetes team or – if you have one – the lead member of the multidisciplinary foot team.

Bed rest is key to offloading a plantar ulcer. Ensure the patient and nursing team understands this important but apparently 'negative' point (it means minimising walking even to the toilet or bathroom).

## After admission

Foot abscesses are common and difficult to diagnose clinically in the profoundly insensitive neuropathic foot. A boggy swelling in the sole of the foot – sometimes communicating to the dorsum – is not always obvious. MRI is helpful for diagnosing collections (**Box 16.1**). There is a tendency now to request MRI scans in a majority of patients – sometimes even before a plain X-ray of the foot. These are complex patients, often with multiple old lesions of the foot and previous amputations. Scans can be difficult to interpret, and it may be 1 or 2 days before you have a formal report, during which time there is a risk that no clinical diagnosis will be made, or that inappropriate treatment is started.

---

**Box 16.1**  Indications for MRI of the diabetic foot

- Suspicion of deep infection – necrotising fasciitis, deep abscess
- As an aid in diagnosing Charcot neuroarthropathy, which usually occurs in the mid-foot, and whose key radiological feature is marrow oedema but osteomyelitis may give a similar appearance. Clinical factors favouring a Charcot process: notably warm skin in the absence of ulceration, oedema
- Establishing the extent of osteomyelitis when plain radiography is equivocal or even negative (**Figure 16.4**)
- Clinical mid-foot and metatarsal fractures that are not clear-cut on plain X-ray

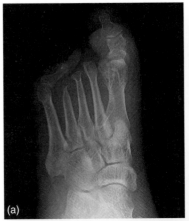

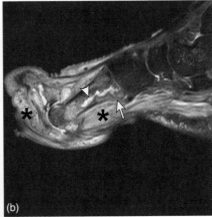

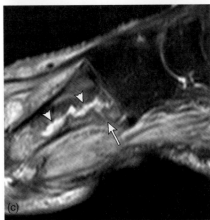

**Figure 16.4** Value of MRI scanning in difficult clinical situations. While (a) the plain radiograph of the left foot is unremarkable for osteomyelitis, the presence of multiple previous amputations and the subluxation at the 5th metatarsophalangeal joint should make you suspicious that there is a new infection. (b) and (c) Fat-suppressed SPAIR sagittal MRI of the same foot as in (a) shows marrow oedema in the first metatarsal, a serpiginous fluid cavity centrally in the shaft (arrowheads), and a small cortical defect (arrow) leading to a sinus track. Soft tissue oedema is marked with asterisks. *Source:* Reproduced with permission of Sergei Kuzmich, Whipps Cross University Hospital.

**Table 16.2** Skeletal infections in diabetes

| Site | Clinical features | Diagnostic methods | Notes |
| --- | --- | --- | --- |
| **Foot digit ('sausage toe', metatarsal head, metatarsophalangeal joint)** | Adjacent ulceration common (sometimes nearly healed) | Sequential plain X-ray | Prolonged course of bone-penetrating antibiotics (e.g. 6–12 weeks) often sufficient. Osteomyelitis of the 1st metatarsophalangeal joint is common (because of frequent underlying ulceration) and rarely heals without surgery. Complex conservative surgery can be successful |

*(Continued)*

**Table 16.2** *(Continued)*

| Site | Clinical features | Diagnostic methods | Notes |
|------|-------------------|--------------------|-------|
| **Mid-foot bones** | Nearly always associated with plantar ulceration | Plain X-ray; MRI | Less likely to heal with prolonged antibiotics. Hyperbaric oxygen therapy possibly of value. Often difficult to distinguish from Charcot neuroarthropathy. Careful surveillance |
| **Vertebral osteomyelitis** (includes vertebral osteomyelitis, discitis, epidural abscess and paraspinal abscess) | Back pain, weakness (paraplegia) and fever. Usually thoracolumbar. Dialysis is a risk factor. Usually haematogenous spread from remote foot ulcer, dialysis lines. Sometimes spontaneous – no primary site identified. | MRI. CRP/ESR usually elevated. Blood culture positive in ~25%. Bone biopsy | Urgent neurosurgical advice, especially if there is paraspinal or epidural abscess. Isolated discitis usually treated with prolonged antibiotics. Always cover MRSA, which is common |
| Septic arthritis | Increased risk in diabetes; knee and hip commonest (as in non-diabetic people). Other joints are more likely to be involved, e.g. shoulder, sternoclavicular, temporomandibular | Early joint aspiration | |

## OSTEOMYELITIS (Table 16.2)

Think of osteomyelitis in any diabetic patient with recent onset bony pain. There is not always a skin infection or ulcer. The earliest radiological signs of osteomyelitis (demineralisation, periosteal reaction and bone destruction) may take 2 weeks or more to develop. However, radiological progression can be very rapid (**Figure 16.5**). Request repeat X-rays every 2 weeks, and ensure you keep in contact with the diabetes or surgical team.

Ensure antibiotic therapy is targeted at bone (microbiology review). In general, distal osteomyelitis affecting the phalanges can often be treated successfully with 12 weeks of appropriate antibiotics (6 weeks may be sufficient). Progressive bone resorption, sometimes with extrusion of bony sequestrum through the skin, is a good outcome here. Osteomyelitic digits presenting as 'sausage toe' are often best managed with surgery, but the remaining foot is so compromised mechanically by the loss the great toe that this situation requires intensive medical treatment before resorting to surgery – unless there is irretrievable skin necrosis (**Figure 16.5**).

In infection of metatarsal and mid-foot bones, 3-monthly cycles of antibiotics guided by sequential MRI scans may be successful, but inevitably some of these cases come to surgery. Hyperbaric oxygen therapy, if available, is indicated as adjuvant treatment in resistant osteomyelitis. Heel ulcers can rapidly progress to osteomyelitis, as the protective fibrofatty tissue in neuropathic patients is thin, and bone infection can proceed alarmingly quickly (**Figure 16.6**).

'Metastatic' osteomyelitis, through haematogenous spread, is fortunately rare, but bear it in mind if there is any distant bony pain – especially spinal pain developing some

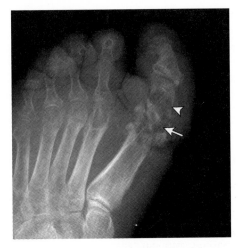

**Figure 16.5** Plain radiograph of the left foot of a diabetic patient, showing extensive osteomyelitic change in the proximal phalanx of the great toe (arrowhead) and the head of the first metatarsal (arrow). There is extensive soft tissue swelling. The state of the skin and subcutaneous tissues will often determine whether the patient should have early surgery. There is a large volume of infected tissue in cases like this, and infection can spread proximally very rapidly. *Source*: Reproduced with permission of Sergei Kuzmich, Whipps Cross University Hospital.

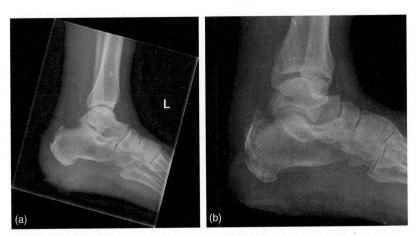

**Figure 16.6** Osteomyelitis can progress rapidly. (a) Normal heel X-ray in a 67-year-old man with Type 2 diabetes, duration 20 years, and a heel ulcer. Very poor control (HbA$_{1c}$ 11%, 97 mmol/mol). Sensitive *S. aureus* on blood culture. (b) 4 weeks later, extensive osteomyelitis despite intensive i.v. antibiotics.

weeks or months after apparent healing of an ulcer or osteomyelitis. Patients must not have eye surgery while there is any infected foot lesion.

In practice, osteomyelitis is nearly always caused by *S. aureus*. Bone biopsy, invasive and difficult to organise, is rarely needed unless you suspect another organism, or there is a poor response to prolonged high-dose anti-staphylococcal antibiotics.

## CHARCOT NEUROARTHROPATHY (Figure 16.7)

Consider a Charcot process in a newly presenting hot, swollen diabetic foot without ulceration (though secondary ulceration occurs: see **Figure 16.7**). It usually presents with painless inflammatory swelling, and the affected foot is several degrees warmer than the contralateral foot. It may be precipitated by minor trauma, resulting in silent metatarsal stress fractures. It is frequently misdiagnosed as gout (unusual in this part of the foot) or 'arthritis'.

It is a rapidly progressing process, always in patients (both Type 1 and 2) with advanced neuropathy, resulting in mostly painless destruction of bones and joints of the foot – characteristically involving the mid-foot, but sometimes the metatarsophalangeal joints and even the ankle. Severe mechanical disruption of the foot occurs if not intercepted – for example, the navicular bone displaces medially and the cuneiforms inferiorly. These may secondarily ulcerate through pressure.

The difficulty is recognising it in the first place: systemic inflammatory markers are unimpressive, so clinical alertness followed by judicious imaging is important. Once diagnosed, the foot needs immediate immobilisation with total contact casting or an Aircast (UK) boot. The diabetes foot team should take over the patient's care. Management is predominantly ambulatory with specialist podiatrists. Specialist surgery can help once the acute process has settled. Bisphosphonates, previously recommended, probably do not affect progression.

## TISSUE VIABILITY TEAM

All hospitals have a specialist tissue viability team. They are formally included in the multidisciplinary foot team structure, but they are in short supply, have other responsibilities, and they may not be able to assess your patients within 24 hours, which is the UK standard. The first port of call is:

## THE MULTIDISCIPLINARY FOOT TEAM

Again, a recent requirement in all UK hospitals. The ideal foot team consists of a diabetologist, a surgeon with an interest in the diabetic foot, a podiatrist, a diabetes specialist nurse, a tissue viability nurse, with *ad hoc* input from physiotherapists and pain management specialists. This is a counsel of perfection, and although highly desirable, many hospitals do not provide this service. But all patients must be referred within 24 hours of admission at least to the diabetes team.

## URINARY TRACT INFECTIONS

Eighty per cent of infections in people with diabetes involve the upper tract, bacteraemia is about four times more likely, and bilateral involvement is more frequent. Treatment should therefore be robust, with antibiotic courses of 7, possibly 14 days, required even in cystitis. Request a renal tract ultrasound scan in everyone. Remember the poorly emptying bladder in patients with longstanding diabetes, who may have neuropathy affecting the bladder (there should be no residual urine volume).

### Bacteria involved
- *E. coli*
- *Proteus* spp.
- *Enterobacter* spp.

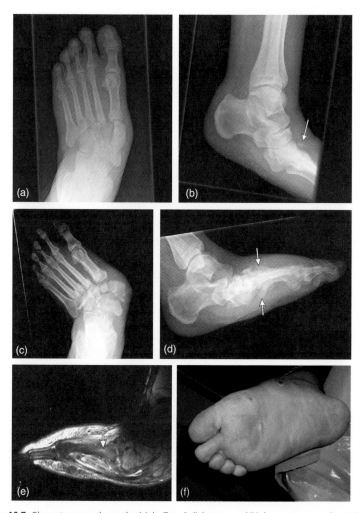

**Figure 16.7**   Charcot neuroarthropathy. Male, Type 2 diabetes, aged 72, known neuropathy. He injured his foot about 7 months before presenting to the specialist podiatry team; he had noticed increasing deformity of the foot, and then developed an ulcer, ultimately 5 cm in diameter over the medial aspect of the tarsometatarsal joint of the great toe. Ulceration with notable foot deformity should alert to a combination of Charcot neuroarthropathy and osteomyelitis. (a) and (b) Anteroposterior and lateral radiographs of the left foot showing the classical radiographic triad of a Charcot foot: (1) dislocation of the 2nd and 3rd tarsometatarsal joints (Lisfranc joint); (2) early destruction of the tarsometatarsal and intermetatarsal joints; and (3) new heterotopic bone formation (arrow). (c), (d): radiographs 6 months later. (c) and (d) Anteroposterior and lateral radiographs with increasing foot deformity with severe dislocation of all the tarsometatarsal joints, progressive destruction of the tarsometatarsal and intermetatarsal joints and exuberant new heterotopic bone formation (arrows). (e) MRI showing early osteomyelitis in the proximal 1st metatarsal indicated by bone marrow oedema (arrow). (f) Male, aged 36, Type 1 diabetes 15 years. He twisted his ankle, but continued to walk on it for 2 weeks because of loss of pain sensation. Typical Charcot foot appearance: flattened arches and medial displacement of the navicular with secondary ulceration from footwear.

- *Enterococcus faecalis*
- *Klebsiella pneumoniae*
- Group B streptococci
- *S. aureus* (perinephric abscess)

## Choice of antibiotic
Consult your local antibimicrobial guidelines

- Uncomplicated cystitis: oral trimethoprim 200 mg bd or nitrofurantoin 50 mg qds for 7 days
- Pyelonephritis: i.v. gentamicin, followed by amoxicillin 1 g every 8 hours
- In the very sick, septic patient: ceftazidime 0.5–1 g every 12 hours, or cefuroxime 0.75–1.5 g every 6–8 hours, or piperacillin-tazobactam 4.5 g every 12 hours

Once fever, systemic symptoms and inflammatory markers have subsided, transfer to oral antibiotics and maintain to make a total of 14 days' treatment.

## Poor response to standard treatment suggests:
- Perinephric abscess (**Figure 16.8**)
- Emphysematous pyelonephritis and cystitis are almost specific to diabetes (**Figures 16.9** and **16.10**). *E. coli* is the commonest organism (70%), but other organisms generating carbon dioxide (through unclear mechanisms) occur: *Proteus mirabilis, Klebsiella pneumoniae,* group D streptococcus, coagulase-negative staphylococcus and more rarely anaerobes such as *Clostridium septicum, Candida albicans, Cryptococcus neoformans* and *Pneumocystis jiroveci*

Both conditions are best imaged with CT; manage them jointly with urologists, radiologists and microbiologists. Emphysematous pyelonephritis is now usually successfully managed medically.

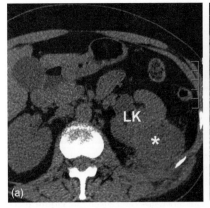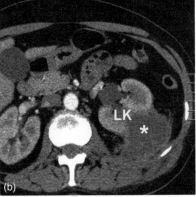

**Figure 16.8** Renal abscess. (a) Unenhanced axial CT image in a diabetic patient presenting with urosepsis shows a hyperdense mass (asterisk) on the left kidney. There is surrounding fat stranding, raising suspicion of an abscess, which is confirmed, (b) in the corresponding enhanced axial CT image. The left renal abscess (asterisk) is shown to be a thick-walled fluid collection with peripheral enhancement and inflammatory change in the surrounding fat. *Source*: Reproduced with permission of Sergei Kuzmich, Whipps Cross University Hospital.

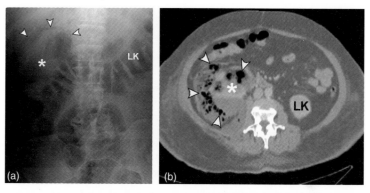

**Figure 16.9** Emphysematous pyelonephritis. (a) Plain abdominal radiograph shows free gas (arrowheads) around the right kidney (asterisk), and outlining it, (b) Corresponding axial CT image confirming pockets of gas (arrowheads) in and around the right kidney (asterisk). Normal left kidney. *Source*: Reproduced with permission of Sergei Kuzmich, Whipps Cross University Hospital.

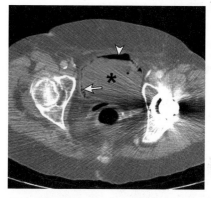

**Figure 16.10** Emphysematous cystitis. Axial pelvic CT image. There are small pockets of gas (arrow) within the wall of the bladder (asterisk), in addition to a more prominent pocket of dependent gas (arrowhead) floating beneath the anterior bladder wall. *Source*: Reproduced with permission of Sergei Kuzmich, Whipps Cross University Hospital.

## ABDOMINAL INFECTIONS

A persistent trap. Symptoms can be subtle and undramatic, sometimes only PUO; autonomic neuropathy with reduced abdominal visceral sensitivity may mask symptoms. The commonest abdominal infection is peritonitis in peritoneal dialysis patients which will be managed by the renal team, but in acute general medicine also consider:

- Emphysematous cholecystitis (polymicrobial – Gram-negatives and anaerobes; **Figure 16.11**)
- Gynaecological infections (I have been caught out by a tiny abscess in the pouch of Douglas, presenting as a PUO without symptoms)
- Bacterial hepatic abscess (uncommon in the UK) – usually *Klebsiella* spp.
- Psoas abscess (see below, musculoskeletal infections)

CT will confirm all these.

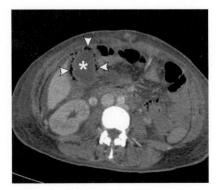

**Figure 16.11** Emphysematous cholecystitis. Axial CT image, showing characteristic small pockets of free gas (arrowheads) in the wall of the gallbladder, which is enlarged and thick-walled. *Source*: Reproduced with permission of Sergei Kuzmich, Whipps Cross University Hospital.

## MUSCULOSKELETAL INFECTIONS

Like abdominal infections, they present atypically, sometimes as a pyrexia of unknown origin, and often with chronic symptoms. Staphylococcus is the usual culprit causing vertebral osteomyelitis (occasionally streptococcus and pneumococcus). *S. aureus* has a particular predilection for the bones of the spine, spreading to form paraspinal abscesses and, as in the foot, requires high levels of suspicion for diagnosis, backed up by plain radiology and MRI, occasionally FDG-PET/CT. Other related infections:

- Septic arthritis (including the sternoclavicular joint)
- Epidural abscess
- Discitis (sometimes associated with vertebral osteomyelitis; **Figures 16.12** and **16.13**)

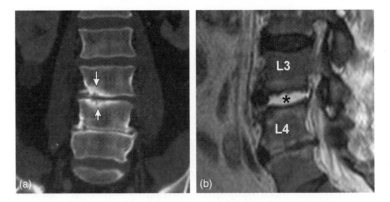

**Figure 16.12** Pyogenic discitis at L3-L4 level. (a) Non-contrast coronal CT image showing sclerosis and erosive changes in the endplates of L3 and L4 (arrows). At an early stage of discitis these changes are unlikely to be detectable on routine radiographs. (b) Corresponding unenhanced T2-weighted close-up image shows that the disc (asterisk) is replaced by intensely bright signal. There are erosive changes in the adjacent endplates, which have an irregular outline. *Source*: Reproduced with permission of Sergei Kuzmich, Whipps Cross University Hospital.

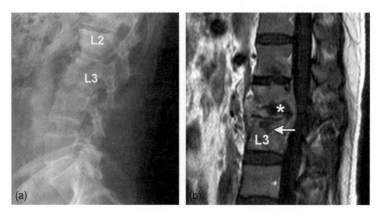

**Figure 16.13** Pyogenic discitis and vertebral osteomyelitis. (a) Lateral plain radiograph showing endplate destruction at L2-L3, more marked in the inferior endplate of L2. (b) Contrast enhanced T1-weighted sagittal MRI reveal osteomyelitic fluid collections in the L2 vertebral body (asterisk) and L3 vertebral body (arrow). *Source:* Reproduced with permission of Sergei Kuzmich, Whipps Cross University Hospital.

- Psoas abscess (classically: fever, flank pain and limitation of hip movement, with positive psoas sign – worsening pain on hip flexion). Primary abscesses are reported in poorly controlled diabetes. Common secondary causes include vertebral osteomyelitis and discitis, genitourinary infections, and less commonly bowel infections and trauma (**Figure 16.14**).
- Pyomyositis, usually affecting the quadriceps; also be aware of diabetic muscle infarction (also known as diabetic myonecrosis, presenting the same way, with thigh pain and swelling, usually in poorly controlled diabetes with established microvascular complications, especially renal)

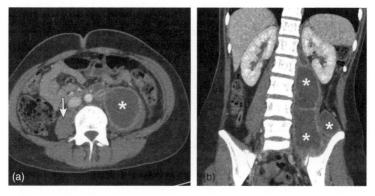

**Figure 16.14** Iliopsoas abscess. (a) Contrast enhanced axial CT image. Left psoas abscess (asterisk) – fluid collection with a thick enhancing capsule and associated enlargement of the left psoas muscle. (b) Corresponding axial CT image showing the lower extent of the iliopsoas abscess (asterisks) as a large thick-walled loculated collection. MRI is best suited for evaluating the extent of spinal (bone) involvement. *Source:* Reproduced with permission of Sergei Kuzmich, Whipps Cross University Hospital.

## CHEST INFECTIONS

It is not known whether diabetes increases the risk of mortality from general community-acquired pneumonias. Pneumococcal and influenzal infections, while not more common (other than bacteraemic pneumococcal infection), are associated with higher morbidity and mortality. Bear in mind the following, more common in diabetes:

- *S. aureus* pneumonia
- Empyema, especially *Klebsiella*, but also *S. aureus* and anaerobes
- *M. tuberculosis*. The WHO recognises diabetes as a risk factor for TB; treatment outcomes are poorer

## UNCOMMON/RARE INFECTIONS THOUGHT TO BE ALMOST SPECIFIC TO DIABETES

- 'Malignant' otitis externa (usually *Pseudomonas aeruginosa*) – severe pain, discharge and hearing loss
- Rhinocerebral mucormycosis – sporadic and rare, and current reports of this invasive fungal infection due to *Mucorales* spp. are mostly from developing countries. I have never encountered a case. It is said to be associated with DKA. Face or eye pain progresses to severe ocular involvement

## POSTOPERATIVE INFECTIONS

- **General surgery, hip replacement surgery**: substantially increased risk of surgical site infection, urinary tract infection and lower respiratory infection
- **Coronary bypass graft**. Leg wounds: increased risk of infection, seroma, dehiscence and haematoma. Sternal wound infections, especially deep infections associated with mediastinitis
- **Spinal surgery**: increased risk of surgical site infections
- **Bariatric surgery**: surprisingly, bariatric surgery in people with diabetes is not associated with an increased risk of operation-related infections (low at around 5%) – nor is preoperative BMI an infection risk factor. This may reflect greater awareness of these risks in extreme obesity, and the fact that glycaemia usually improves dramatically immediately after surgery

### Further reading

Ertegrul BM, Lipsky BA, Savk O. Osteomyelitis or Charcot neuro-arthropathy? Differentiating these disorders in diabetic patients with a foot disorder. *Diabet Foot Ankle.* 2013;4. PMID: 24205433.
Peters EJ, Lipsky BA. Diagnosis and management of infection in the diabetic foot. *Med Clin North Am.* 2013;97:911–46. PMID: 23992901.

# PART 4
# Insulin and non-insulin agents

# 17 Variable Rate Intravenous Insulin Infusion (VRIII, 'sliding scale' – UK; insulin drip – USA)

**Top tip**

Consider alternatives to intravenous insulin infusions: they are time-consuming for nursing staff and generally difficult for patients.

**Key points**

- Definition: A slow continuous intravenous infusion of soluble/fast-acting insulin, running variably at 0.5–8 U/hr, for control of blood glucose levels in patients with persistent hyperglycaemia not associated with hyperglycaemic emergencies, who are not eating and for whom subcutaneous fast-acting insulin cannot be used
- The rate of infusion is changed usually according to hourly CBG measurements. If CBG levels are stable, testing frequency can decrease to 2-hourly or 4-hourly
- Give an intravenous infusion of glucose at the same time to prevent hypoglycaemia
- A separate infusion of rehydrating fluids (0.9% NaCl, Hartmann's, PlasmaLyte) will be needed in the acutely unwell patient or someone who is not drinking
- Use insulin infusions with common sense and wherever possible try to think of a safe and effective alternative, even though it may result in more work for you in the short term

## INDICATIONS FOR VRIII (Table 17.1)

**Table 17.1** Good and not such good uses for VRIII

| Consider VRIII | Don't consider VRIII |
| --- | --- |
| Managing BG levels in patients who are unable to eat and whose BG levels are consistently >15 mmol/L or thereabouts. Priority is patients taking insulin before admission, but all patients with uncontrolled BG levels should have VRIII initially – but for as short a time as possible while other strategies are considered | In well patients with transient elevations of BG – unless the patient is ketotic |
| Perioperatively (see **Chapter 27**) | In patients where a simple increase in non-insulin agents or insulin would be more useful in the medium term |
| In the recovery phase of DKA or HHS, when ketosis and chemistry are corrected, but when patients may be nauseated or otherwise unwilling/unable to eat | In patients who were previously treated for severe hypoglycaemia who have 'rebound' hyperglycaemia (see **Chapter 26**) |
| Parenteral feeding (usually ICU) | |

*The Hands-on Guide to Diabetes Care in Hospital,* First Edition by David Levy.
© 2016 John Wiley & Sons, Ltd. Published 2016 by John Wiley & Sons, Ltd.

Most hospitals have a protocol for VRIII. They differ in detail, but the principles are the same:

**1.** Intravenous insulin acts quickly, and more predictably than subcutaneous insulin; the dose can be adjusted hourly (or more often if need be) to maintain target inpatient CBG levels (7–10 mmol/L)
**2.** Insulin dose adjustments are made in response to instantaneous blood glucose readings; more sophisticated algorithms take into account prior rates of change of BG, but in practice the simpler system works well
**3.** Most hospitals have integrated documents for prescribing insulin (traditionally 50 units Actrapid in 50 mL 0.9% NaCl in a 50 mL syringe to run via a syringe driver, but any soluble or rapid-acting analogue insulin is suitable) and a suggested starting insulin scale, a glucose monitoring chart, and a mechanism for prescribing a new scale
**4.** Run intravenous glucose at the same time, for example, 100 mL 5% glucose hourly
**5.** The numerical scales vary, and their origins obscure[1]

## Changing scales

Some hospitals suggest different scales that escalate infusion rates across the BG range if the default scale does not give adequate control. In practice, the problem is often concentrated at the higher CBG levels on the initial scale, and usually responds to increasing the rates at higher levels rather than uniformly increasing them (**Table 17.2**).

**Table 17.2** Example of a change to an i.v. insulin scale when it is more difficult to correct high BG levels than lower ones

| CBG (mmol/L) | Default scale (U/hr) | Proportionately increased scale (U/hr) | Skewed increased scale (U/hr) (often more effective) |
|---|---|---|---|
| 0–4.0 | 0 | 0 | 0 |
| 4.1–7.0 | 1 | 2 | 1 |
| 7.1–11.0 | 2 | 4 | 3 |
| 11.1–16.0 | 3 | 6 | 4 |
| 16.1–21.0 | 5 | 8 | 6 |
| >21 | 6 | 10 | 8 |

This means that where possible, construct your own revised scale taking into account the behaviour of blood glucose levels under conditions of high and low insulin doses. In conditions of insulin resistance (e.g. acute pancreatitis, **Chapter 15**) or high glucose loads (e.g. artificial feeding, **Chapter 28**) insulin infusion rates may need to be substantially increased at higher levels of CBG (e.g. 10–16 U/hr).

## Continue long-acting insulin

Long-acting background subcutaneous insulin should be continued if patient was admitted on it – give the same insulin in the same dose at the same time of the day (usually once daily at bedtime or in the morning). This is good practice in all patients taking insulin, but particularly so in Type 1 patients, where it will protect against ketosis if intravenous insulin is discontinued – for example, while an i.v. line is re-sited.

---

[1] They probably originated in the far-off days of colour-coded BM (Boehringer-Mannheim) strips, whose readings were grouped into ranges: 0–4, 4–7, 7–11, 11–16, 16–21 and higher.

### Fluids to run at the same time

'Flip-flop' regimens are in widespread use, where 5% glucose is infused if BG is lower than some arbitrary number, for example, 12 or 14 mmol/L, and replaced with 0.9% NaCl if BG exceeds the arbitrary number. It is generally unsatisfactory:

**1.** It is difficult for nursing staff
**2.** In someone who is nil by mouth it can result in inadequate rehydrating fluids
**3.** The threshold for changing infusion fluids has no evidence base

It is more logical to use the following, according to whether or not the patient needs rehydration and whether or not they are eating. (Table 17.3).

**Table 17.3** Blood glucose control and i.v. rehydration according to the clinical situation

|  | Needs rehydration | Adequately rehydrated |
|---|---|---|
| **Not eating** | (5 or 10% glucose +VRIII) + PlasmaLyte | 5 or 10% glucose + VRIII |
| **Eating** | Usual diabetes treatments + PlasmaLyte | No i.v. needed |

### Alternative glucose infusions where there is a risk of fluid overload

In patients with heart failure, where you want to minimise i.v. fluids, use for example 10% glucose, infused at 50 mL/hr, or 20% glucose at 25 mL/hr. Where there is central venous access in critically overloaded patients, 50% glucose can be given by syringe driver at 10 mL/hr.

# 18 Converting from VRIII to subcutaneous insulin

**Top tip**

Do not total the previous day's intravenous insulin dose and give in divided doses subcutaneously once the VRIII finishes. If the patient is new to insulin, use the guides in **Chapters 22** and **23** – 0.5 U/kg/day is generally safe.

There is a widespread practice of using the most recent total 24-hour intravenous insulin requirement to convert unit for unit into a 24-hour subcutaneous insulin dose in patients not previously using insulin. While there is a broad correlation between i.v. and s.c. insulin requirements using standard VRIII regimens, it cannot be reliably translated safely into an individual's insulin requirement. Using this relationship would be especially hazardous in converting newly presenting DKA patients treated with 10% glucose and high-dose fixed-rate insulin at 6 U/hr (these patients are likely to move into 'honeymoon' or partial temporary remission shortly after diagnosis when insulin requirements may fall dramatically).

Several US studies have recommended only 40–50% of the previous day's intravenous insulin requirements to be given as basal insulin with supplementary mealtime insulin based on CHO counting at mealtimes. Patients in these studies are generally obese (BMI >30, weight 90–100 kg), so the resulting doses – 35–50 units – seem reasonable and compatible with the safe conservative calculation of a total daily insulin dose of 0.5 U/kg.

One study found that *any* post-operative conversion from intravenous to subcutaneous insulin was poor at maintaining target BG levels, but that fewer adjustments were needed in those started on a weight-based insulin regimen. Safety – especially minimising the risk of severe hypoglycaemia – is the primary concern.

Patients already taking insulin can be converted to their pre-admission regimen, with a general reduction in doses of ~20% to allow for a temporary decrease in appetite and food intake.

*The Hands-on Guide to Diabetes Care in Hospital,* First Edition by David Levy.
© 2016 John Wiley & Sons, Ltd. Published 2016 by John Wiley & Sons, Ltd.

# 19 Writing safe insulin prescriptions

## Top tip

Insulin is usually at or near the top of the list of drugs involved in prescribing errors in hospital (often omission – which may be hazardous and lead to ketoacidosis in ketosis-prone patients).

## Key points

- SLOW DOWN AND THINK when you write an insulin prescription, especially when you're on emergency duty at night: errors can be serious, possibly fatal
- Write insulin up as soon as possible, and as a priority (see **Chapter 7**)
- Generic insulin isn't available in the UK: insulin is always prescribed by brand name (e.g. 'NPH insulin' cannot be dispensed or administered; prescribe Humulin I, Insulatard or Insuman Basal)
- Wherever you can, confirm the exact name of the patient's insulin: unless the insulin has been obtained out of the UK, it WILL be among the list in **Chapter 20**
- Insulin is NEVER a 'prn' drug
- Give insulin as a 'stat' dose ONLY when it replaces a dose that has been omitted
- Avoid using 'stat' doses of insulin to 'correct' 'high blood glucose levels'
- Write insulin names in block capitals
- Nearly all insulin is presented at a concentration of 100 U/mL, so do not risk confusing this with a dose – omit the concentration. The long-acting analogue Tresiba has a double-strength preparation (U200, 200 U/mL), as does Humalog, but they are only available in a prefilled pen, so there is no possibility of prescribing or administration error. The same applies to a U300 (300 U/mL) preparation of Lantus (Toujeo)
- If you do not have charts with preprinted 'units', do not abbreviate dosages to U or IU: write 'units' in full
- In biphasic insulin preparations, the suffix 25, 30 or 50 does not refer to a dose but the proportion of fasting-acting insulin. However, patients could be taking, for example: NovoMix 30, 30 units before breakfast
- Unless you are certain about the injection device the patient uses, focus on prescribing the insulin in the correct doses; ward staff and diabetes specialist nurses will help out with the device
- Drug regulatory authorities now require unique names for new insulin preparations. While this reduces the risk of confusion between similar-sounding preparations (e.g. Actrapid and NovoRapid) the names convey little to signify that they are actually insulin preparations, nor their intended duration of action

*The Hands-on Guide to Diabetes Care in Hospital,* First Edition by David Levy.
© 2016 John Wiley & Sons, Ltd. Published 2016 by John Wiley & Sons, Ltd.

# 20 Insulin preparations in the UK (BNF section 6.1.1)

**Top tip**

Twenty per cent of inpatients have diabetes, and about a quarter will be taking insulin. Learn the exact names of the most frequently used insulin preparations (see **Table 20.1**).

The number of insulin preparations available is now smaller than ever as manufacturers 'rationalise' their product ranges. Only about 10 insulin preparations are in common use in the UK, of which 7 are so-called 'analogue' insulins, human insulin molecules modified to make them either shorter-acting or longer-acting than their biosynthetic human counterparts. Prescribing practice will often differ markedly between different hospitals for 'historical' reasons. This means that insulin preparations you have become familiar with may not be available when you move to your next job. But your patients still need their insulin.

In *practice*, the differences between the older biosynthetic human insulins (from the 1980s) and analogue insulins (from the 1990s onwards) are limited, and of no practical significance in the acute hospital setting. It is therefore permissible and safe to substitute insulin preparations in the emergency situation (see **Chapter 22**).

**Table 20.1** shows all the insulin preparations available in the UK in the middle of 2015. Note that Actrapid, the default human soluble insulin in UK hospital practice, is not used by patients in the community as it is not available in cartridge or pen form. However, it can of course be used as a substitute s.c. soluble insulin as an emergency (see **Chapter 23**). Generic (biosimilar) analogue insulins, especially glargine (Lantus) will be introduced over the next few years as their patents expire.

## BACKGROUND INFORMATION

About 80% of UK patients use analogue insulins, but Type 2 patients are increasingly being encouraged to use human preparations, as they are in all clinical respects similar to the comparable analogues. A tiny number (they are nearly all long-standing Type 1 patients) use animal (pork) insulin (Hypurin preparations), and may be unhappy to take human or analogue preparations. If their pork insulin isn't available, then discuss short-term human insulin substitution.

Intravenous insulin is conventionally given as Actrapid (human soluble [fast-acting] insulin). It is 'always' available, but any short-acting insulin (**Table 20.1**) can substitute. Actrapid is no longer available in cartridge or pen form in the UK, so it is not used in ambulatory patients.

The majority of patients in the UK use cartridge pens (refillable or disposable) to give their insulin. Your duty as a prescriber is to focus on the insulin itself and not the specific device (but for details, see **Chapter 33**).

*The Hands-on Guide to Diabetes Care in Hospital,* First Edition by David Levy.
© 2016 John Wiley & Sons, Ltd. Published 2016 by John Wiley & Sons, Ltd.

**Table 20.1** Insulin preparations available in the UK (2015) The font size is an approximate representation of how often they are used in the community setting. A: analogue insulins (modified human insulins, shaded boxes); H: synthetic recombinant human insulins.

| Short-acting | Basal insulin (intermediate or long-acting) | Biphasic insulin mixtures (fixed mixtures of short- and intermediate-acting) |
| --- | --- | --- |
| • Taken 10–30 minutes before meals | • Taken at bedtime (or morning, or twice daily about12 hours apart) *independent of mealtimes.* | • Taken twice or three times daily before meals |
| • Clear insulin | • Human preparations are cloudy, analogues are clear | • Cloudy |
| NovoRapid (aspart, A) Humalog (lispro, A) Humulin S (H) Insuman Rapid (H) Apidra (A) | Lantus (glargine, A) Levemir (detemir, A) Humulin I (H) Insuman Basal (H) Insulatard (H) Tresiba (degludec, A) Abasria (biosimilar glargine) (A) | NovoMix 30 (A) Humulin M3 (H) Humalog Mix25 (A) Humalog Mix50 (A) Insuman Comb (15, 25 and 50) (H) Ryzodeg (Tresiba/NovoRapid) (A, clear insulin) |

## NOTES ON INDIVIDUAL INSULIN PREPARATIONS

### Short-acting insulins
Usually given three times a day before meals (ideally 10–30 minutes before eating). They are likely to be ineffective and predispose to hypoglycaemia if given after meals.

In the UK, NovoRapid and Humalog are by far the commonest mealtime insulins. You will encounter the others much less frequently – in both Type 1 and Type 2 patients.

In the pressured ward environment, mealtime insulin doses are not always given correctly before meals. Write clear instructions in BLOCK CAPITALS exactly when you intend them to be given e.g. '15 minutes before meals'.

### Basal insulin
Provided by long-acting insulin preparations, usually given at bedtime (22:00 in hospital), occasionally in the morning, sometimes twice daily, approximately 12 hours apart.

The current sound recommendation is that usual basal insulin is continued in hospital, especially in Type 1 patients, as a prophylaxis against ketosis, in case fast-acting insulin (s.c. or i.v.) is discontinued for any reason.

A common regimen for Type 2 diabetes is basal insulin at bedtime, combined with a variety of non-insulin agents during the day.

In Type 1 diabetes, basal insulin is nearly always combined with fast-acting mealtime insulin, usually three times a day (though breakfast-avoiders and students often only have two doses, lunch and evening meal)

In the UK, Lantus (commonly referred to by its generic name 'glargine') and Levemir are the commonest basal insulins, but increasingly, Type 2 patients (and some Type 1) are using older human preparations, especially Humulin I (I = isophane, otherwise known as NPH insulin). The very long-acting analogue Tresiba is not yet in widespread use, and either of the other long-acting analogues could substitute.

## Biosimilar insulins

The insulin equivalent of generic drugs. Several are in development for launch after the patent on analogue insulins expire. For example, Abasria (Lilly/Boehringer Ingelheim) is a biosimilar glargine.

## Biphasic insulins

Mixtures of fast-acting and intermediate-acting insulin in fixed proportions (usually 25% or 30% fast-acting). They are most commonly used in Type 2 patients. Like short-acting insulins, they must be given before meals, and never after a meal or between meals.

Some children and young people prefer the convenience of twice-daily biphasic insulin (before breakfast and evening meal); increasingly, overweight Type 2 patients will use three times daily biphasic mixtures, especially the 50% fast-acting preparation Humalog Mix50.

*Caution: distinguish between the various Humalog preparations.* Take care to distinguish between Humalog (fast-acting), and Humalog Mix25 and Humalog Mix50 (biphasic) insulin in prescriptions. Inadvertent prescribing of Humalog where Humalog Mix was intended is unlikely to cause problems, but vice versa there is a risk of hypoglycaemia between meals because of the additional and substantial intermediate-acting component.

## Non-UK insulin preparations

Occasionally patients will be admitted taking insulins not available in the UK, some of which may have different names. Look carefully at prescriptions or preferably the insulin vials/cartridges/packages (**Table 20.2**). Note US names of biphasic insulins put the proportion of intermediate-acting insulin first, not the proportion of fast-acting insulin.

**Table 20.2** Insulin preparations you may encounter in use by overseas patients.

| Name | UK name |
| --- | --- |
| NovoLog | NovoRapid |
| NovoLog Mix 70/30 | NovoMix 30 |
| Humulin R [R = regular = soluble] | Humulin S [S = soluble] |
| Humulin N [N = NPH] | Humulin I [I = isophane] |
| Humalog Mix75/25 | Humalog Mix25 |
| Humalog Mix50/50 | Humalog Mix50 |
| Humulin R U-500 [high concentration 500 U/mL] | Not prescribable in the UK |

All have identical preparations available in the UK with different brand names. U-500 Humulin R is not prescribable in the UK.

# 21 Commonly used insulin regimens

> **Top tip**
>
> Gain confidence in using insulin in your patients by focusing on the patterns of insulin use throughout the day and the reasons for them.

**Insulin regimen** = pattern of subcutaneous insulin administration through the day and night. The doses required are almost infinitely variable, so decisions on starting doses and subsequent titration are separate from determining the regimen.

Consider insulins in three groups (see **Chapter 20**), shown modified below (**Table 21.1**). To simplify it, only the 10 major insulin preparations are included here as examples.

**Table 21.1.** Major insulin preparations in the UK, grouped according to their action

| Group 1<br>Basal insulin (intermediate<br>or long-acting) | Group 2<br>Short-acting | Group 3<br>Biphasic insulin mixtures<br>(fixed mixtures of short- and<br>intermediate-acting) |
|---|---|---|
| *Background insulin usually taken once a day, often bedtime. Slow-acting, so no need to take at a mealtime* | *Taken before meals* | *Taken two or three times daily before meals. Background insulin is supplied by the intermediate-acting component* |
| Lantus (glargine)<br>Levemir (detemir)<br>Humulin I<br>Tresiba (degludec) | NovoRapid (aspart)<br>Humalog (lispro)<br>Humulin S | NovoMix 30<br>Humulin M3<br>Humalog Mix25, Humalog Mix50 |

## BASAL INSULIN (GROUP 1; Figure 21.1)

### Type 1 diabetes

Basal insulin mimics background pancreatic insulin secretion and suppresses ketosis. Although usually taken at bedtime, the morning suits some patients, especially if there has been nocturnal hypoglycaemia. Twice-daily basal insulin, taken about 12 hours apart (e.g. evening meal and first thing in the morning), is also used. Nearly all Type 1 patients need additional mealtime insulin (usually two or three injections daily), but there is a small but important group with very longstanding Type 1 diabetes where blood glucose control is erratic, with a tendency to hypoglycaemia with even tiny doses of fast-acting insulin, and basal insulin alone is the safest option, even though postprandial glucose control is poor.

*The Hands-on Guide to Diabetes Care in Hospital,* First Edition by David Levy.
© 2016 John Wiley & Sons, Ltd. Published 2016 by John Wiley & Sons, Ltd.

## Type 2 diabetes

Basal insulin in Type 2 diabetes has a different rationale from Type 1 diabetes. It helps control fasting hyperglycaemia, resulting from failure of endogenous insulin to suppress hepatic glucose levels, especially overnight. In the early stages of insulin-treated Type 2 diabetes, basal insulin is frequently combined with daytime oral agents (metformin, sulphonylureas, gliptins, flozins, glitazone; **Chapter 24**) with or without an injected long-acting GLP-1 analogue. Most of these, apart from metformin, affect post-prandial glucose levels. The different physiology (and differences in body weight) in Type 1 and Type 2 diabetes means that Type 1 patients often need much smaller doses of basal insulin to control fasting levels – for example, 20–30 units (sometimes lower), compared with 40–80 units.

### Variant

'Basal-plus': basal insulin, often together with non-insulin agents, plus one prandial dose of fast-acting insulin taken with the largest meal of the day, usually dinner. This can be progressively extended to cover other meals where prandial glucose control isn't satisfactory.

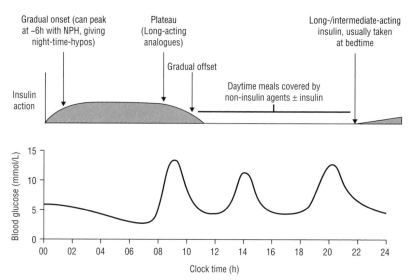

**Figure 21.1** Basal insulin in diabetes, superimposed on a typical 24-hour glucose profile. The long-acting analogues glargine and levemir have a longer action than the intermediate-acting isophane (NPH) insulins, but *in practice*, they are used more for their smoother nocturnal profile with a lower risk of night-time hypoglycaemia than their extended reach; degludec, however, is genuinely an ultra-long-acting insulin.

## BASAL-BOLUS REGIMEN (GROUP 1 + GROUP 2; Figure 21.2)

### Type 1 diabetes

The prototype multi-dose insulin (MDI) regimen, consisting of basal insulin at bedtime and short-acting insulin (bolus) given three times daily before meals. It is the easiest and most flexible regimen to start in a hospital patient newly requiring insulin (see

**Chapter 22)**. A large majority of Type 1 patients worldwide use this regimen – but it does not guarantee good glycaemic control.

Variants
- Omitting breakfast insulin (basal insulin, especially long-acting analogues, will continue to act until around lunchtime); omitting lunch or evening meal insulin in people doing exercise in the afternoon or evening, respectively
- Additional doses taken with substantial carbohydrate-containing snacks
- Many Type 1 patients now do some form of carbohydrate counting, in order to adjust their mealtime insulin doses to the amount of carbohydrate taken. DAFNE – Dose Adjustment for Normal Eating – is one of several formal educational programs for educating Type 1 patients in adjusting insulin doses

### Type 2 diabetes
Patients frequently graduate to basal-bolus regimens if basal overnight insulin with daytime non-insulin agents fails to control blood glucose. However, control is probably no better in most patients than with other insulin regimens.

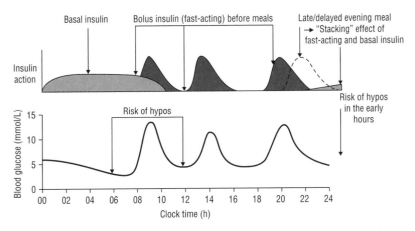

**Figure 21.2** Basal-bolus regimen. Widely used in both Type 1 and Type 2 diabetes. In ambulatory practice hypoglycaemia tends to occur, (a) in the middle of the night or just before waking as a result of the basal insulin taken the previous night, and (b) before lunch because of physical activity superimposed on breakfast insulin (and possibly the tail end of the basal insulin).

## BIPHASIC (FIXED-MIXTURE) INSULIN REGIMENS – Usually Two Times Daily Before Breakfast and Evening Meal, Sometimes Three Times Daily (GROUP 3; Figure 21.3)

### Type 1 diabetes
Often used in schoolchildren and young people, especially if they are unable to take insulin more often than twice daily and wish to avoid lunchtime injections. Control is usually less good than with a multi-dose regimen, particularly over the lunch period, which is not covered by fast-acting insulin, and overnight.

## Type 2 diabetes

Similar to Type 1 diabetes, though the human mixtures (e.g. Humulin M3) tend to be used more than the analogue mixtures. Often combined with metformin and other non-insulin agents.

## Variant

Three-times daily biphasic insulin, sometimes a 30/70 mixture, but usually a 50/50 mixture (e.g. Humalog Mix50) – taken before each main meal. On occasion this can be supplemented with basal bedtime insulin to correct fasting hyperglycaemia – a modified basal-bolus regimen.

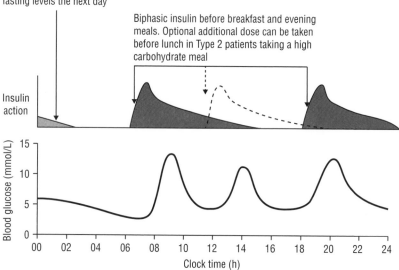

Figure 21.3 Biphasic insulin. Still occasionally used in Type 1 diabetes, and widely in Type 2 (often with metformin and other non-insulin agents, and usually as a step-up treatment from basal insulin + non-insulin agents). Because there is no fast-acting insulin at lunchtime, control in the middle of the day in Type 1 patients is often poor. Three-times daily biphasic insulin with 50% fast-acting component (Humalog Mix50, Insuman Comb50) is becoming more widely used in Type 2 patients who eat a substantial lunch. A generally unsuccessful variant in Type 1 students averse to injecting in the middle of the day consists of biphasic insulin with breakfast, fast-acting insulin with the evening meal, and basal insulin at bedtime – three different insulin preparations.

## INSULIN PUMP (CONTINUOUS SUBCUTANEOUS INSULIN INFUSION, CSII; Figure 21.4)

A device for continuously administering fast-acting analogue insulin subcutaneously via a cannula into the fat of the abdominal wall as a variable basal dose, given at about 0.3–1.0 U/hr, supplemented by larger bolus doses of the same insulin to cover meals and snacks. Used only in Type 1 diabetes. Regimens are highly variable and flexible, and are designed to mimic a basal-bolus regimen. Used carefully and with intensive education, insulin pump treatment can improve well-being and reduces the risks of severe hypoglycaemic reactions and DKA.

Insulin pumps are increasingly used in Type 1 patients, so you are more likely to encounter them in hospital. Ask the diabetes team to review.

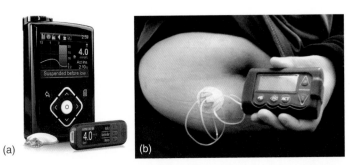

(a)      (b)

**Figure 21.4** Insulin pump. (a) Advanced (sensor-augmented) insulin pump (MiniMed 640G®). Centre: pump. Lower left: continuous glucose monitoring device inserted at a separate site from the pump cannula; glucose results are continuously available for the user. Lower right: remote control device. Minimed 640G is a registered trademark of Medtronic Ltd and the image is the property of Medtronic Ltd. (b) MiniMed Paradigm pump (Medtronic). This is an example of an older generation of pump, still in widespread and successful use. The delivery set and cannula are usually placed in the subcutaneous tissue of the abdomen.

# 22 Emergency subcutaneous insulin regimens

**Key points**

- Starting patients on insulin is not very difficult, but is avoided like poison by most trainees
- Where possible, consult with the inpatient diabetes team, who will be more adept at doing this than you. But there will be occasions when it will be helpful to patients to start subcutaneous insulin without delay
- Key aims are to avoid severe hyperglycaemia (CBG consistently >15 mmol/L), ketosis in Type 1 or insulin-deficient Type 2 patients and hypoglycaemia (symptoms or CBG <4 mmol/L)

## Situations
- Newly diagnosed Type 1 patients no longer requiring intravenous insulin infusion if no specialist input is available (e.g. weekends, public holidays)
- Type 2 patients admitted with hyperglycaemia and ketosis (= insulin deficiency), who are best treated with insulin in the first instance
- Type 2 patients in poor control on maximum non-insulin agents, especially if they are not overweight

## SCENARIO 1: NEW BASAL-BOLUS INSULIN (Multiple Dose Insulin, Three Injections of Fast-acting Preprandial Insulin, One Dose of Long-acting Insulin at Bedtime)

You can start any patients on this, but it is mandatory in Type 1 patients, to ensure there are no periods without insulin where ketosis might develop (especially in patients who have just recovered from DKA).

### 1. Calculate total daily insulin requirement
- Weigh the patient                                                        e.g. **76 kg**
- Starting total daily insulin requirement = 0.5 units of insulin/kg body weight **38 units**
- A thin newly diagnosed Type 1 patient may be especially sensitive to insulin, so reduce to 0.4 or even 0.3 U/kg

---

*The Hands-on Guide to Diabetes Care in Hospital,* First Edition by David Levy.
© 2016 John Wiley & Sons, Ltd. Published 2016 by John Wiley & Sons, Ltd.

2. **Give approximately 50% of this dose as long-acting basal insulin given at bedtime**                                                    **20 units**

Use any long-acting insulin available on the ward. You are most likely to have access to:

- Lantus
- Levemir
- Humulin I

3. **Give the remaining insulin (18 units) as mealtime fast-acting insulin**

Give higher doses with lunch and evening meal as they are likely to contain higher carbohydrate amounts.

For example:

- Before breakfast                                             **4 units**
- Before lunch                                                 **6 units**
- Before evening meal                                          **8 units**

Use any available fast-acting insulin:

- NovoRapid
- Humalog
- Humulin S
- (avoid Actrapid unless no others are available; it is not available in pens and cartridges in the UK, so is not a practicable insulin for discharge)

You don't need to specify any injection device in your prescription: just concern yourself with the doses.

## SCENARIO 2: NEW TWICE-DAILY BIPHASIC INSULIN (TYPE 2 PATIENTS)

1. **Calculate total daily insulin requirement**
   - Weigh the patient                                          e.g. **76 kg**
   - Starting total daily insulin requirement = 0.5 units of insulin/kg body weight  **38 units**
2. **Give approximately 2/3 of this dose before breakfast**        **25 units**
3. **Give the remaining 1/3 before evening meal**                  **14 units**

Use any available mixture containing 25% or 30% fast-acting insulin:
- NovoMix 30
- Humalog Mix25
- Humulin M3

**Caution:** these calculations are approximations, and patients will differ in their responses, especially in the setting of an acute illness. Ensure meticulous daily 7-point CBG testing, and review these results every day with the aim of adjusting insulin doses to achieve CBG 7–10 mmol/L.

Adjust relevant insulin doses by 2 units each, or in patients on higher doses, e.g. >30 units, by 10%. Review insulin doses every day.

**7- point CBG testing**: before meals, 1½ – 2 hours after meals and at bedtime.

# 23 Substituting insulin preparations in the emergency setting

**Key points**

- Omitting insulin doses is potentially hazardous
- Insulin should never be omitted because the patient's own insulin preparations are not available or known, for whatever reason
- There will always be a safe substitute insulin preparation available
- Do not start a VRIII unless you really cannot source an appropriate alternative in time for the next due subcutaneous injection

Substituting insulin preparations that are not immediately available is not a situation you will often find yourself in, but it is important, especially in Type 1 patients, who may become ketotic if a single injection is missed. The usual scenario is a patient you see in the emergency department who has forgotten to bring their insulin with them and documentation of their usual insulin regimen. Do your best to find out the names of the intended insulin preparations. Simple questions will help you identify at least the *type* of insulin, and possible the exact preparation (see **Figure 7.3**). Ensure insulin is written up before the patient is transferred to another department or ward.

Reinstate the original preparations as soon as they are confirmed and available. Time-consuming but important: discuss with the patient, carers/relatives, general practitioners and ward pharmacist.

## DISCUSSION WITH PATIENTS

Insulin is a highly personal medication, and wherever possible explain the importance of substituting insulin, but with reassurance that you will reinstate the patient's usual insulin as soon as possible. Memory-impaired patients, especially if they are unwell, may not be able to tell you accurately the names of their usual insulins, and occasionally patients will recall insulin preparations they have used in the past, but which they may not have been taking for several years. It is particularly hazardous to transcribe half-recalled names of insulin into a prescription record.

## SUBSTITUTION

Use the information in **Table 23.1**.

*Doses*. Nearly all patients who give their own insulin injections will know the doses. In the very small number of patients who know the frequency and type of their insulin, but not the number of units they take, see **Chapter 22**. Start with a total daily dose of 0.5 U/kg body weight.

*The Hands-on Guide to Diabetes Care in Hospital*, First Edition by David Levy.
© 2016 John Wiley & Sons, Ltd. Published 2016 by John Wiley & Sons, Ltd.

**Table 23.1** Suggestions for first- and second-line subcutaneous insulin substitutions for use in an emergency until the patient's usual insulin can be reinstated

| Insulin to be substituted | First-line replacement | Second-line and subsequent replacements |
|---|---|---|
| **Fast-acting insulins** | | |
| Humulin S | Actrapid (vial only) | NovoRapid, Humalog |
| NovoRapid | Humalog | Apidra, Actrapid, Humulin S |
| Humalog | NovoRapid | Apidra, Actrapid, Humulin S |
| Hypurin Porcine Neutral | – | Humulin S, Insuman Rapid |
| **Intermediate- and long-acting insulins** | | |
| Insulatard | Humulin I | Insuman Basal |
| Humulin I | Insulatard | Insuman Basal |
| Hypurin Porcine Isophane | – | Humulin I, Insulatard |
| Lantus | Levemir | Humulin I, Insulatard |
| Levemir | Lantus | Humulin I, Insulatard |
| Tresiba | Lantus | Levemir |
| Abasria | Lantus | Levemir |
| **Biphasic mixtures** | | |
| Humulin M3 | NovoMix 30, Humalog Mix25 | Humalog Mix25 |
| NovoMix 30 | Humalog Mix25 | Humulin M3 |
| Humalog Mix25 | NovoMix 30 | Humulin M3 |
| Humalog Mix50 | – | Humulin M3, Insuman Comb 50 |

# 24 Non-insulin agents (BNF sections 6.1.2.1-3)

## Key points

- Know about metformin and the sulphonylureas (SU)
- Be aware of the other agents (**Box 24.1**), and ask for advice if you are unfamiliar with them
- Apart from SUs, and metformin in mild-to-moderate CKD, omitting other agents because they are not immediately available is unlikely to result in severe hyperglycaemia in the short term

**Box 24.1**  Non-insulin agents

- **Metformin**
- **Sulphonylureas** (SU)
- **DPP4 inhibitors** (gliptins)
- **GLP-1 analogues** (s.c. injections)
- **Pioglitazone** (glitazone)
- **SGLT2 inhibitors** (flozins)

There are many classes of diabetes drugs (**Box 24.1**), used in multiple combinations, often with insulin as well. Broadly speaking, the more agents, the more likely is glycaemic control to be poor. You should know in outline what the classes of medication are and how they work, but the only ones you need to know in detail for inpatients are metformin and the SUs.

Your dealings with metformin will be limited to withholding it, at least temporarily, or decreasing the dose. The fear is lactic acidosis, though cases are extremely rare. If you are concerned, measure lactate: the current view on limited overdose data is that plasma lactate <3.5 mmol/L is safe.

Metformin accumulates in renal impairment, leading to an increased risk of lactic acidosis, but is not itself nephrotoxic – despite a widely held view, sometimes irresponsibly conveyed to patients. However, abruptly stopping metformin in patients with stable renal impairment can cause rapid and marked deterioration in glycaemic control. Wherever possible, tail down the dose over a few days and watch CBGs.

Sulphonylureas work quickly (within 24–48 hours), so are of value in some hyperglycaemic states. All remaining drug groups are designed for community use and work much more slowly – many may not have a useful effect on BG level for a few weeks.

## METFORMIN

### Discontinue metformin

- In AKI
- If eGFR <30 mL/min

*The Hands-on Guide to Diabetes Care in Hospital,* First Edition by David Levy.
© 2016 John Wiley & Sons, Ltd. Published 2016 by John Wiley & Sons, Ltd.

- In systemic sepsis
- In acute heart failure
- One scheduled dose before an investigation using contrast; reinstate 24 hours afterwards if eGFR >60 mL/min
- One scheduled dose before surgery; reinstate when eating and eGFR >60 mL/min

**Minimise metformin dose in CKD 3 (30–59 mL/min)** to maintain CBG 9–13 mmol/L (HbA$_{1c}$ ≅ 8.5% (69); Table 24.1).

**Table 24.1** Metformin dosing in CKD

| eGFR level (mL/min) | Action |
| --- | --- |
| ≥60 | No renal contraindication |
| 45–59 | Continue metformin |
| 30–44 | Lower metformin dose e.g. halve, or half-maximal dose (no more than 1 g/day) |
| <30 | Discontinue |

*Source:* From Lipska et al. 2011.

## If you discontinue metformin:

- Intensify blood glucose monitoring, for example, fasting levels and one or two measurements during the day, and start insulin when BG levels are >15 mmol/L
- Metformin predominantly affects fasting glucose levels, so start with basal overnight insulin
- Restart it as soon as it is safe to do so, or make alternative plans for ensuring BG control when the patient goes home. They may become severely hyperglycaemic without metformin – which is as powerful as any other agent in diabetes

**Rule of thumb:**  start bedtime (2200) Humulin I or Insuman Basal at the same numerical dose as fasting blood glucose (e.g. 14 U if FBG 14 mmol/L), and increase daily by 2 U (or 10% at doses higher than 30 U) until target BG reached.

**Maintain metformin unless there are other contraindications in:**
- Uncomplicated ACS (**Chapter 13**)
- Steroid-treated patients (**Chapter 29**)

### Metformin and lactic acidosis (Box 24.2)

**Box 24.2**  Characteristics of lactic acidosis in patients taking metformin

- (History of metformin administration)
- Blood pH <7.0
- Very high lactate level (>15 mmol/L)
- Large anion gap (>20 mmol/L)
- Renal insufficiency (eGFR <45 mL/min or serum creatinine >180 μmol/L)

Metformin-induced lactic acidosis is Type B (nonhypoxic). It is exceptionally rare, but life-threatening, and usually occurs in patients with moderate–severe CKD and a severe acute illness who have continued taking metformin, often in high doses (Kalanter-Zadeh et al., 2013). Hypoglycaemia at presentation is rare, because metformin does not stimulate peripheral glucose uptake. Toxic levels of metformin can cause acute pancreatitis. Get urgent ICU advice; venovenous haemofiltration treats the severe acidosis and AKI and also removes metformin. Compared with lactic acidosis from other causes, the prognosis is good.

## SULPHONYLUREAS (SU)

### Agents most commonly used in the UK

- *Gliclazide.* Maximum effective dose is probably 80 mg bd (=120 mg m/r form). Maximum licensed dose is 320 mg daily (though the dose-response relationships for SUs are weak, and increasing the dose above 160 mg/day in the hospital setting is unlikely to be helpful: prepare your patient and yourself for starting insulin)
- *Glimepiride.* A once-daily SU, taken in the morning. Dose range: 1–6 mg daily, maximum effective dose probably 4 mg daily
- *Glibenclamide* (a long-acting agent, now little used, mostly because of concern about hypoglycaemia). It is still widely used out of the UK, often in its branded form (Daonil), dose range usually 2.5-15 mg daily, twice daily above 10 mg
- *Repaglinide* is a short-acting SU-like drug taken in a dose of 0.5–4.0 mg up to three times daily before main meals

### Discontinue SU

- If patient is nil by mouth
- In acute hepatic dysfunction (SUs are hepatically metabolised)

### Maintain sulphonylurea

- In steroid-treated patients (**Chapter 29**)
  - Brief trial of SU (e.g. gliclazide 80 mg bd or glimepiride 2 mg mane) if BG <15, but be prepared to rapidly change to insulin
  - Patients already on SU: don't bother increasing beyond these doses, and move to insulin (maintain SU but observe for hypoglycaemia 2–4 hours after dose)

### SU-induced hypoglycaemia

Common, and can be significant (most patients report symptoms with SUs at 3.0 mmol/L – this is classified as serious hypoglycaemia, so if any hypoglycaemia is reported or detected, reduce dose if possible). In outpatients taking SUs, hypoglycaemia characteristically occurs 2–4 hours after a morning dose, that is mid- to late-morning, but most hypoglycaemic reactions in hospital occur – worryingly – in the early hours of the morning (see **Figure 24.1**). Note that insulin-induced hypoglycaemia shows an identical pattern, peaking in the early morning.

### Interactions

Possibility of haemolysis in patients with G6PD deficiency
Hypoglycaemia with some antibiotics. In decreasing order of likelihood:

- Clarithromycin (nearly fourfold increased risk)
- Levofloxacin
- Co-trimoxazole
- Metronidazole
- Ciprofloxacin

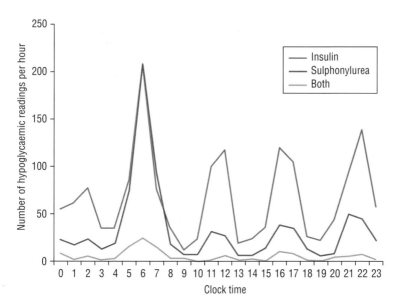

**Figure 24.1** Hypoglycaemic reactions by clock time in hospitalised UK patients taking insulin, SU or combination insulin/SU. Hypoglycaemia: CBG ≤3.9 mmol/L. Note the major peak in the early hours of the morning with prominent further peaks between meals, after dinner, and in the early hours. *Source*: Reproduced with permission of Rajendran et al. 2014.

## OTHER CLASSES OF MEDICATION

### DPP4 inhibitors (gliptins)
Sitagliptin, saxagliptin, linagliptin, vildagliptin, alogliptin

- Modestly increase insulin secretion by inhibiting breakdown of the native incretin hormone GLP-1
- Once-daily dosage (most are licensed for use with or without dose reduction in renal impairment; **Table 24.2**)
- They are safe in mild-to-moderate hepatic impairment (Child-Pugh Class A and B). Discontinue in severe hepatic impairment, where insulin is likely to be the safest treatment option
- Slow onset of action and relatively weak antihyperglycaemic agents (HbA$_{1c}$ reduction ~0.5%). They have no place in acute treatment of hyperglycaemia
- Concerns about increased pancreatitis risk have not been substantiated

### Pioglitazone (glitazone, PPARγ agonist)
Used now only in small numbers of patients after cardiac concerns in the mid-2000s led to the withdrawal of rosiglitazone. You can continue pioglitazone unless there is heart failure or peripheral oedema. Discontinuing pioglitazone has an unpredictable effect on BG levels. Patients will probably not need insulin treatment in the short term, but watch CBGs carefully, and on discharge remember to let the patient's GP know that you have recommended discontinuing it.

**Table 24.2** Dosing of DPP4 inhibitors (gliptins) in renal impairment

| DPP4 inhibitor | Full dose | Dose reductions in renal impairment |
|---|---|---|
| Sitagliptin (Januvia) | 100 mg mane | eGFR 30–50 mL/min – 50 mg<br>eGFR <30, ESRD (dialysis) – 25 mg |
| Saxagliptin (Onglyza) | 5 mg mane | Moderate/severe renal disease – 2.5 mg<br>ESRD – do not use |
| Linagliptin (Trajenta) | 5 mg mane | Dose unchanged in all degrees of renal impairment, including (with caution) in dialysis |
| Vildagliptin (Galvus) | 50 mg bd | All degrees of renal impairment and ESRD – 50 mg daily |
| Alogliptin (Vipidia) | 25 mg mane | eGFR 30–60 mL/min – 12.5 mg mane<br>eGFR 15–30, dialysis – 6.25 mg mane |

## GLP-1 analogues (subcutaneous injection via disposable injection pen)

- Synthetic analogues of the incretin hormone GLP-1, which stimulate insulin secretion without themselves causing hypoglycaemia. Small dose-response range
- Exenatide (Byetta, twice daily before breakfast and evening meal), liraglutide (Victoza, once daily, independent of mealtimes), lixisenatide (Lyxumia, once daily, independent of mealtimes)
- Bydureon/Bydureon Pen (once weekly), Trulicity (dulaglutide, once weekly)
- Combination long-acting basal insulin (degludec) and liraglutide in fixed escalating dosage steps (Xultophy)
- Discontinue if there are any acute GI symptoms, especially nausea or vomiting
- Given using disposable pens. Patients can confuse these agents with insulin. They are often used in combination with insulin. Licensed mostly with basal (long-acting) insulin, apart from dulaglutide which is licensed with multi-dose insulin, many patients successfully use them with a variety of insulin regimens

### SGLT2 inhibitors (flozins)
The newest drug class. Dapagliflozin (Forxiga), canagliflozin (Invokana), empagliflozin (Jordiance) and several others in development

- Inhibit renal glucose reabsorption. Once-daily dosage
- Increased risk of urinary tract infection and thrush. Discontinue if admitted with these or they develop during admission. Discontinue in patients with AKI or hypovolaemia; do not use in combination with diuretics
- Canagliflozin (100 mg daily) and empagliflozin (10 mg daily) are licensed at these lower doses in patients whose eGFR falls from >60 mL/min to 45–60 mL/min

## References

Kalanter-Zadeh K, Uppot RN, Lewandrowski KB. Case records of the Massachusetts General Hospital. Case 23-2013. A 54-year-old woman with abdominal pain, vomiting, and confusion. [Metformin toxicity and its management]. *N Engl J Med.* 2013;369:374–82. PMID: 23841704.

Lipska KJ, Bailey CJ, Inzucchi SE. Use of metformin in the setting of mild-to-moderate renal insufficiency. *Diabetes Care.* 2011;34:1431–7. PMID: 21617112.

Rajendran R, Kerry C, Rayman G; MaGIC Study Group. Temporal patterns of hypoglycaemia and burden of sulfonylurea-related hypoglycaemia: a retrospective multicentre audit of hospitalised patients with diabetes. *BMJ Open.* 2014;4(7): e005165.

# PART 5
# Blood glucose management on the wards

# 25 Managing patients you are asked to see with high blood glucose levels

**Key points**

- This is one of the commonest requests you will encounter from the wards
- Don't action a high blood glucose level without a proper (albeit brief) clinical assessment of the patient and without reviewing the last couple of days' blood glucose monitoring results in conjunction with the drug chart
- Think longer term than the next hour – difficult though that might be when you're pressurised to 'do something'
- Don't write up 'stat' s.c. doses of soluble insulin; while such regimens are in use in the UK, in general they encourage treating numbers and not patients and their clinical problems. They are rarely of value and can cause severe hypoglycaemia

Up to 20% of patients in hospital at any time have diabetes. Many of them were in poor glycaemic control before admission; control is likely to be further compromised by intercurrent infection, steroids, enteral feeding and inconsistent administration of prescribed medication.

## Numerical example

Take a patient in moderately poor control, for example, $HbA_{1c}$ 9% (75 mmol/mol). The upper 95% confidence interval for random blood glucose levels at this $HbA_{1c}$ is 14.0 mmol/L; that is, 1 in 20 measurements in an *otherwise well* patient will be >14 mmol/L. Blood glucose levels in the high teens and low twenties are common in hospital practice in otherwise clinically stable patients.

## THE PATIENT WITH CBG >20 mmol/L (see Table 25.1)

**Table 25.1** A general approach to patients with high blood glucose levels.

| CBG chart | Clinical scenario | Approach |
| --- | --- | --- |
| Isolated ↑CBG on a background of reasonable control | • Ensure diabetes medication was given on time and in the prescribed dose(s). Ask gently about recent sugary or high carbohydrate food or drink <br> • Was the patient hypoglycaemic earlier in the day (CBG <4 mmol/L, treated or not)? | • If non-insulin agents were omitted, no action other than monitor CBG 2-hourly <br> • If insulin was omitted, give about 30% of the prescribed dose, and request 2-hourly CBG <br> • Gentle education <br> • Counter-regulation and administered glucose. Allow to settle: don't start VRIII (risks repeat hypoglycaemia) or 'stat' insulin doses |

*(Continued)*

*The Hands-on Guide to Diabetes Care in Hospital,* First Edition by David Levy.
© 2016 John Wiley & Sons, Ltd. Published 2016 by John Wiley & Sons, Ltd.

**Table 25.1** *(Continued)*

| CBG chart | Clinical scenario | Approach |
|---|---|---|
| CBG climbing over >6–12 hours on background of reasonable control | • Emerging illness, especially infection?<br><br>• Early hyperglycaemic emergency?<br>• Sometimes together<br>• Recent steroids<br><br>• Diabetes medication omitted on several occasions | • History, brief exam, focused investigations (laboratory glucose, FBC, CRP, Cr+elec, cultures)<br>• Exclude early hyperglycaemic emergency, especially if CBG in high twenties: if urinary ketones ≥1+ or capillary ketones >1.5 mmol/L, check venous gases; if urinary ketones negative, calculate plasma osmolarity<br>• Exclude early hyperglycaemic emergency, brief VRIII until next dose due. Ensure that medication is or will be written up properly |
| CBGs erratic, but frequently high | • Common in sick, hospitalised patients (multifactorial, often on a background of poor overall glycaemic control) | • Exclude any immediately treatable problem (new infection), review recent blood test results (WBC, CRP for developing infection, AKI) and manage accordingly. Otherwise, record your observations of poor control and request team to review soon (and involve the diabetes team, especially if there is hypo- as well as hyperglycaemia) |
| High CBG at the same time on more than one day | • Common, often reflecting change in timing and content of hospital meals | • Analyse the problem. If you are the patient's doctor, increase medication or insulin to avoid your colleague being called the next day for the same reason. If the patient is under another team's care, make concise suggestions in the notes about your recommendation |

In some patients you will not find a specific reason, but always do a brief formal clinical assessment (for infection and early hyperglycaemic emergency) and do not automatically 'treat' with an intravenous insulin infusion. If CBG measurements are recorded consistently at the same high number (e.g. 27.8 mmol/L = 500 mg/dL) request an urgent laboratory blood glucose, because the actual reading may be >27.8 mmol/L.

## VRIII AND 'STAT' DOSES OF SOLUBLE INSULIN

See **Chapter 17** for guidance on appropriate use of VRIII.

Giving small 'stat' doses of soluble insulin in automatic response to a 'high' blood glucose level is widely practised, and some hospitals have guidelines for it. See below for some personal comments, but until we have continuous glucose monitoring for all inpatients with reliable warnings of hypoglycaemia, the hazards of unexpected hypoglycaemia are likely to outweigh any benefits of temporarily reducing a high number. Where there is unexpected hyperglycaemia in response to a new infection or other medical or surgical illness, then intercepting early hyperglycaemic emergencies, while fully assessing and treating the underlying problem will involve definitive treatment, either with a VRIII or as part of managing early HHS or DKA.

### Comment

The automated and elided process ('high blood glucose' → 'something must be done' → stat dose of soluble insulin) is an example of uncritical medicine-by-numbers – but more serious, it causes considerable anxiety, disruption and discomfort to patients, almost never warranted.

One patient, of which I have direct knowledge, died as a result of a 'stat' dose of Actrapid 6 units given uncritically to 'correct' a one-off CBG of 21 mmol/L in the early hours of the morning; she was an elderly person, but in fact had longstanding and highly unstable (brittle) Type 1 diabetes. She died of hypoglycaemia around 6 hours after the stat dose; she had already been given her usual bedtime dose of Lantus, and presumably BG levels were already falling by the time the corrective dose was given. She had been admitted overnight because she couldn't get back home late in the evening after suffering a simple accidental arm fracture.

The perceptual psychology is interesting, and presumably reflects an inbuilt tendency to regard a spot biochemical measurement as lying on a horizontal, stable, line, against any common sense or statistical likelihood. (Interestingly, we are all taught that in the case of physiological measurements, e.g. BP or urine output, we must consider rates of change, rather than instantaneous measurements, before initiating treatment; in general this teaching is successful, so it is curious that biochemical measurements are not assessed in the same way.) The likelihood of the patient having a genuinely flatlining BG

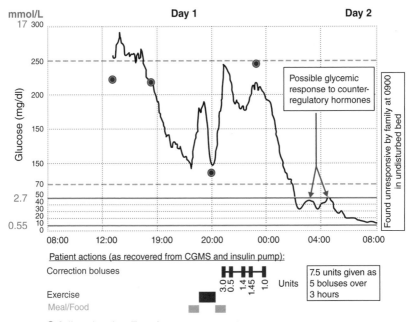

**Figure 25.1** Retrospective continuous glucose monitoring system analysis of 'dead in bed' syndrome. The patient gave himself a total of 7.5 units of fast-acting insulin in 5 boluses over the course of 3 hours between about midnight and 4-00 am. Peak BG just before midnight was 12.2 mmol/L, but only 2 hour later was 1.7 mmol/L. Around 4-00 am two minor peaks in BG levels (up to 2.7 mmol/L) probably represented counter-regulatory responses, but circulating insulin levels were still presumably significant after the boluses and over the next 3 hours BG fell to almost undetectable levels. Note the general BG instability in this Type 1 patient, which isn't unusual: the previous day BG levels had fallen in a nearly identical way from 17 mmol/L to 5 mmol/L over a similar period. BG levels almost never 'flatline' in Type 1 diabetes, or probably in Type 2 either. Before considering prescribing a 'stat' dose of, for example, Actrapid insulin 6 units, reflect on the possible direction and speed of BG changes, which are unknowable based on a single BG estimation. *Source*: From Tanenberg et al. 2010, reproduced with permission from the American Association of Clinical Endocrinologists.

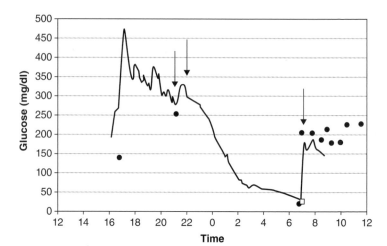

**Figure 25.2** Severe hypoglycaemia recorded in a hospitalized patient with type 1 diabetes, 1 day after orthopaedic surgery (blinded continuous glucose monitoring system, Medtronic). Two insulin preparations, long-acting and rapid-acting analogues were taken at 21:00 pm. The patient was found unresponsive at 07:00 am with a CBG of 1.0 mmol/L. There was a prompt response to intravenous glucose. *Source*: From Joseph et al. 2009, reproduced by permission of the publishers.

is extremely low. In many cases the blood glucose will be rising, in which case a small dose of soluble insulin is unlikely to be of value, especially if the patient has Type 2 diabetes and the usual array of insulin-resistance-inducing hospital conditions; in other cases, it will be falling, perhaps precipitously, with the same token dose in an insulin-sensitive patient accelerating the fall to dangerous hypoglycaemia.

## Literature care report
There is a case report of this phenomenon in a Type 1 patient with difficult-to-control Type 1 diabetes, recently started on an insulin pump (continuous subcutaneous insulin infusion, **Chapter 21**). At the time of his death he was using a continuous glucose monitoring system, the data from which was subsequently downloaded, and tracked accurately his blood glucose levels in the hours before his hypoglycaemic death (**Figure 25.1**). Another near-miss captured on CGMS in a Type 1 patient after orthopaedic surgery has also been reported (**Figure 25.2**). The lesson is clear.

## References
Joseph JI, Hipszer B, Mraovic B, Chervoneva I, Joseph M, Grunewald Z. Clinical need for continuous glucose monitoring in the hospital. *J Diabetes Sci Technol*. 2009;3:1309–18. PMID: 20144385.

Tanenberg RJ, Newton CA, Drake AJ. Confirmation of hypoglycaemia in the "dead-in-bed" syndrome, as captured by a retrospective continuous glucose monitoring system. *Endocr Pract*. 2010;16:244–8. PMID: 19833577.

# 26 Management of acute hypoglycaemia on the ward

## Top tip

Hypoglycaemia, especially if severe (e.g. BG <2.0 mmol/L) is a serious event and may be life-threatening.

## Key points

- Hypoglycaemia is CBG <4.0 mmol/L, regardless of whether symptoms are present or not
- Severe hypoglycaemia is CBG <3.1 mmol/L
- Life-threatening hypoglycaemia is usually CBG <2.0 mmol/L
- Increasing severity and number of episodes of hypoglycaemia are associated with an increased risk of death in the year after discharge from hospital (though causality not established)
- Because of its seriousness, you need to be able to deal with all cases of hypoglycaemia yourself:
  - Treat (many hospitals now have hypoglycaemia kits on the wards)
  - Assess cause of hypoglycaemia by looking at drug treatment chart and CBG monitoring chart together
  - Adjust treatment to lower the risk of recurrent events
- Asymptomatic low CBG levels – treat with oral glucose
- Severe hypoglycaemia requires parenteral treatment followed by oral glucose once patient has recovered
- You are responsible for taking reasonable action to ensure that recurrent hypoglycaemia is avoided
- Non-diabetic hypoglycaemia seems to be increasingly common

You will nearly always be called to do something about a 'high CBG', which is not usually of clinical significance, but unless hypoglycaemia results in impaired consciousness, you are unlikely to be called. However, hypoglycaemia is of itself hazardous and patients with the most severe degrees of hypoglycaemia in hospital (even a single episode) have a poor prognosis for life in the year after discharge.

*The Hands-on Guide to Diabetes Care in Hospital,* First Edition by David Levy.
© 2016 John Wiley & Sons, Ltd. Published 2016 by John Wiley & Sons, Ltd.

## MILD/ASYMPTOMATIC/BIOCHEMICAL HYPOGLYCAEMIA (CBG <4.0 mmol/L)

Patients in poor control may be quite symptomatic at these levels; patients in very good long-term control may have no symptoms.

Important: inform patient that they have low BG, enquire after symptoms, if any, and discuss with them the importance of treating it before they develop symptoms; some patients will not regard CBG <4.0 as hypoglycaemic, so this is a good opportunity to reinforce education.

### ORAL TREATMENT (Figure 26.1)

Measure CBG after 15 minutes and give further CHO if <7 mmol/L (remember that CBG may have been falling – perhaps rapidly – at the point when mild hypoglycaemia was detected).

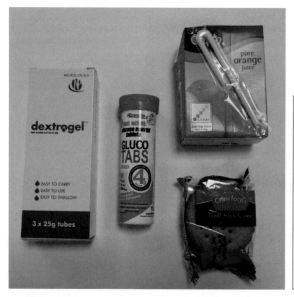

- 200 mL fruit juice
- Pack of 3 biscuits
- 1 × 25 g tube of dextrogel
- 5 × glucose tablets (4 g each)
- 100 mL Lucozade or equivalent glucose sports drink

Liquid meal supplements (e.g. Ensure) are not suitable because they contain isomaltulose, and peak glycaemia occurs nearly 1 hour after that of sucrose.

**Figure 26.1** Treatment of mild hypoglycaemia (~20 g carbohydrate).

### SEVERE HYPOGLYCAEMIA (BG <3.1 mmol/L)

**The presentation is very variable:**
- In sick people in hospital there may be no clinical features (especially if there have been recurrent hypoglycaemic episodes)
- Acute hemiparesis
- Fit

Urgent action is needed and parenteral treatment is safer in people who may have an impaired swallow.

## PARENTERAL TREATMENT (Figure 26.2)

**Glucagon** (which raises blood glucose level mostly through hepatic glycogenolysis), given intramuscularly using a standard kit, is safe and effective, though it acts slower than intravenous glucose. Use it freely where there is likely to be delay in establishing intravenous access – which is common in these sometimes combative people.

It will be less effective in the poorly nourished patient with poor hepatic glycogen stores, and in sulphonylurea-induced hypoglycaemia, where prolonged infusions of 10% glucose are often needed.

### Intravenous glucose

- 50% glucose is much less used now because it is hypertonic and can cause severe tissue necrosis if it extravasates.
- Give 100 mL 20% glucose by rapid i.v. infusion over 5 minutes.

### Sulphonylurea-induced hypoglycaemia

- Glucagon is of no value (will further stimulate insulin secretion)
- Treat with 20% glucose, followed by 10% glucose infusion which may need to continue for 24 hour if the hypoglycaemia was caused by glimepiride, gliclazide or glibenclamide.

### Follow-up

- Give substantial carbohydrate – 2–3 slices of bread or several biscuits
- Record CBG every 30 minutes until consistently in the comfort zone, 7–10 mmol/L
- Maintain patient's usual insulin unless this episode is consistent with a pattern of insulin-induced hypoglycaemia – reduce culprit (preceding) insulin doses

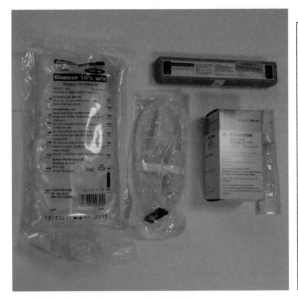

*If the patient can swallow:*
- Treat as above with oral agents

*If consciousness is impaired, give parenteral treatment:*
- Glucagon 1 mg i.m. if venous access is likely to be delayed

Then:
- 100 mL 20% glucose i.v. rapidly into a large peripheral vein (remember air inlet if you use an infusion bottle)
- Follow up with 100 mL/ hr 10% glucose until CBG consistently >7 and patient is fully conscious and able to take oral carbohydrate

**Figure 26.2** Treatment of severe hypoglycaemia.

- If the patient is due a meal shortly after an episode of severe hypoglycaemia – ensure that some insulin is given, for example, 30% of the intended dose
- Severe hyperglycaemia after an episode of severe hypoglycaemia is not uncommon (a combination of endogenous counter-regulation and administered glucose and glucagon). Perversely, this is sometimes 'corrected' by an i.v. insulin infusion (VRIII). Consider the physiological illogicality and potential foolhardiness of giving additional insulin to someone who has just suffered the effects of insulin excess. This advice is repeated for emphasis in **Chapter 17**
- Get advice and help if the patient continues to be hypoglycaemic

## NON-DIABETIC HYPOGLYCAEMIA

Surprisingly common: there are many causes. Consider:

- Factitious administration (by self or others) of insulin or other hypoglycaemic agents, perhaps less common than crime novels and celebrity cases would suggest
- Hypocortisolism (primary adrenal disease, secondary ACTH deficiency): metastatic disease of the adrenals (breast, lung primary) and panhypopituitarism from pituitary metastasis, sometimes isolated (breast, lung) are distressingly common
- Severe malnutrition
- Malabsorption
- Pancreatic disease (chronic pancreatitis, atrophic/calcific pancreatic disease in patients with longstanding Type 2 diabetes; see **Chapter 15, Figure 15.4**)
- Advanced metastatic carcinomas
- Terminal illness in non-cancer cases
- Classic textbook causes – in practice very uncommon: IGF-producing tumours

### Emergency investigations

- Urgent serum samples for C-peptide and insulin if CBG <~2.5 mmol/L. Use a standard biochemistry container (yellow), but take the specimen personally to the laboratory to ensure that it can be separated and frozen without delay. Take a confirmatory venous plasma glucose as well
- Random plasma cortisol

### Treatment

- i.v. 10% glucose, 100 mL/hr, and increase rate to maintain CBG >4
- If there is unremitting hypoglycaemia, start octreotide 50 mcg s.c. 8 hourly, and urgently contact the diabetes/endocrine team

### Further reading

Joint British Diabetes Societies. The hospital management of hypoglycaemia in adults with diabetes mellitus (revised September 2013). Available from: www.diabetologists-abcd.org.uk/JBDS/JBDS.htm (accessed on 1 February 2015).

# 27 Perioperative management of elective surgery

**Top tip**

Hypoglycaemia is probably as harmful as or more than moderate hyperglycaemia in the perioperative period – aim for 7–10 mmol/L.

**Key points**

- CBG variability is very high in both Type 1 and Type 2 diabetes. Never make a decision on cancelling or postponing surgery on the basis of a single random BG measurement
- Patients likely to be starved briefly (only one missed meal): avoid VRIII (insulin infusion) wherever possible and modify usual diabetes medication
- Patients likely to miss more than one meal: plan VRIII
- Patients with Type 1 diabetes require particularly careful planning to avoid ketosis and hypoglycaemia

## PATIENTS SUITABLE FOR DAY-CASE SURGERY

- In reasonable control (HbA$_{1c}$ ≤8.5%, 69 mmol/mol)
- Diet-treated, or using oral agents with or without injected treatment, so long as:
  - They have the first slot on the operating list
  - They are self-managing (can take their own diabetes medication and can monitor CBGs)
  - They can be escorted home and will not be left alone overnight

## POORLY-CONTROLLED PATIENTS

- HbA$_{1c}$ >8.5% (69 mmol/mol), that is, random capillary measurements consistently >9–14 mmol/L
- Many hospitals have guidance for managing these patients and attempting to bring them into better control for major elective surgery
- Unless there are specific community resources for preoperative input, use the inpatient diabetes team rather than referring back to primary care. Patients often require intensive education and significant changes to their diabetes treatment, requiring frequent contacts for dose titration, especially insulin

*The Hands-on Guide to Diabetes Care in Hospital,* First Edition by David Levy.
© 2016 John Wiley & Sons, Ltd. Published 2016 by John Wiley & Sons, Ltd.

- If you identify patients on the ward or in surgical outpatients for whom elective surgery is planned, refer directly to the hospital diabetes team, especially the DSNs
- Be realistic. Scrutinise historical HbA$_{1c}$ values. If persistently high over several years, *and* the patient is known to a specialist diabetes team, they are unlikely to be able to work glycaemic magic in 6 weeks when they haven't been able to do so over the past many years. Meticulous perioperative control and judicious changes to insulin regimen and some education may have long-term benefits in diabetes nurse-naive patients
- Repeated delay and postponements may be more harmful and distressing to the patient than poor glycaemia with sensible explanation of risks, for example, increased postoperative and wound infections

## ADMISSION THE NIGHT BEFORE SURGERY

- Guidelines advise not to admit the night before surgery, and maintaining blood glucose levels overnight probably does not reduce perioperative complications if prior control is poor
- However, ensuring stable blood glucose levels may avoid unnecessary last-minute cancellations and anxiety, especially in Type 1 patients, where an evening admission to set up a VRIII a few hours before surgery is reasonable. The practical difficulty of arranging such an admission in the UK is no reason not to do your best to attempt it
- The problem, especially in Type 2 patients, may not just be poor glycaemic control – electrolytes, BP and renal function are likely to be abnormal as well (acknowledging that these factors should have been managed before admission)

## MANAGEMENT OF DIABETES MEDICATION

### 1 Patients likely to have a short starvation period – maximum one missed meal

### a. Oral agents with or without injected GLP-1 analogues (exenatide, liraglutide, lixisenatide, dulaglutide)

Usual medication the day before admission
- Modified-release metformin if taken twice daily: Although the risks of taking an evening dose of m/r metformin are very low (possible hypoglycaemia), suggest taking the whole day's metformin dose in the morning in the few days before admission
- Bydureon/Bydureon Pen (exenatide)/Trulicity (dulaglutide) – long-acting (weekly) GLP-1 analogues. Do not take an injection within 3 days of an operation
  i. *Morning and afternoon surgery*
  Omit morning oral agents and injected GLP-1 analogue (some exceptions are proposed by JBDS guidelines, but these are counsels of perfection). Normal evening medication if the patient is still in hospital.
  ii. *Evening surgery*
  Not recommended, of course, but patients requiring surgery for infected feet are often put back to the end of the routine list. These are often sick patients, usually already on insulin, and are best managed with VRIII for the fasting period before the operation and until the next morning.

## b. Insulin (Table 27.1)

- Do everything you can to ensure that insulin-taking patients (Type 1 and Type 2) are listed for morning surgery
- Day before admission: no need for any dosage changes
- Always check CBG on admission
- If patients are taking an unfamiliar regimen, for example insulin combined with new or unfamiliar agents, ask diabetes team for advice.

**Table 27.1** Pre-operative insulin management

| Insulin regimen | Day before admission | On the day of surgery (morning surgery assumed) | Comments |
|---|---|---|---|
| **Basal insulin**<br>Long-acting, usually taken at bedtime (e.g. Lantus, Levemir, Humulin I, Insuman Basal)<br><br>If taken in the morning, reduce dose by 1/3 | No dose change – but scrutinise fasting CBG levels. If 4–6, then reduce evening dose by 1/3 to avoid risk of hypoglycaemia during the morning | Check CBG on admission | Maintain insulin dose throughout admission, but withhold any other non-insulin agents |
| **Twice-daily insulin**<br>Usually biphasic mixtures (e.g. NovoMix 30, Humalog Mix25 or 50) | No dose change (but see above, especially if patients have late evening meal) | Give half the usual morning dose, leave evening dose unchanged (unless patient not yet eating) – will probably need overnight VRIII | Withhold any other non-insulin patients |
| **Multiple-dose insulin (basal-bolus)**<br>Usually long-acting at bedtime and fast-acting insulin before meals (e.g. Humalog, NovoRapid), but increasingly three times daily biphasic mixture (e.g. Humalog Mix50, especially in overweight Type 2 patients) | Reduce basal insulin by 1/3 (as above) if fasting levels are 4–6 | Keep any basal insulin unchanged. Omit morning and lunchtime doses.<br><br>Take normal breakfast dose if pm surgery (but reduce by 1/3 if fasting level is 4–6) | Withhold any other non-insulin agents |

## 2 Major surgery – patients likely to miss more than one meal

- VRIII always required
- Discontinue VRIII as soon as possible, but don't do so after about 15:00, because s.c. insulin may not be administered reliably, and overnight CBG monitoring may not be reliable

- Omit the preoperative high-glucose drinks (part of the Enhanced Recovery Programme) in patients treated with insulin

## INTRAVENOUS FLUIDS

Insulin must be given with a continuous glucose infusion to prevent hypoglycaemia. In general VRIII should run with 5% glucose + KCl 10 mmol/L at 100–125 mL/hr. JBDS recommends 'dextrose-saline' with KCl, but many hospitals in the UK no longer use it. Glucose given with the VRIII and a separate infusion of Hartmann's or PlasmaLyte for fluid status is sound. 'Flip-flop' regimes are unhelpful (**Chapter 17**).

### Further reading

Joint British Diabetes Societies. Management of adults with diabetes undergoing surgery and elective procedures: improving standards (April 2011). Available from: www.diabetologists-abcd.org.uk/JBDS/JBDS_IP_Surgery_Adults_Full.pdf (accessed on 24 August 2015)

# 28 Enteral feeding

**Key points**

- Anticipate rapid swings of blood glucose levels in patients starting on enteral feed. Enteral feeds are based on isomaltulose, which is isocaloric with sucrose. Though absorbed more slowly than sucrose, glycaemic excursions can still be dramatic after starting feeds
- There is no reason to use diabetes-specific formulations, which have only marginal glycaemic benefits
- The majority of patients will require insulin treatment, but use s.c. insulin wherever you can, as enteral feeding is likely to be medium- or long-term
- Discuss the feeding regimen with the specialist dieticians, and tailor the insulin regimen accordingly; watch carefully for changes in regimen
- Targets for glycaemic control are similar to those of any hospitalised patient, between 7 and 10 mmol/L
- Involve the diabetes team early on

Glycaemic control in enterally fed patients is often easier to achieve than in free-feeding patients because of the regularity of the regimen, but glycaemic control in these sick patients is still often very poor, exposing them to increased infection risk. Despite the lower glycaemic index of isomaltulose in the feeds compared with sucrose, glycaemic excursions can still be quite dramatic (see **Figure 28.1**).

## Non-insulin agents, including oral hypoglycaemics (Chapter 24)

Non-insulin agents do not act quickly, so do not initiate them in enterally fed patients. If there are no contraindications to their use, there is no need to discontinue them. SUs should be given only at the start of a feed, and to avoid post-feed hypoglycaemia should not be used unless the feed lasts >12 hours.

DPP4 inhibitors (gliptins) have weak glycaemic effects and can be discontinued, and pioglitazone could also be withdrawn except where there is evidence of a good previous glycaemic benefit. The injected GLP-1 analogues can be continued, but do not initiate these agents as they often cause nausea and sometimes vomiting in the early stages of treatment.

**Metformin** can be continued if there are no contraindications. Unfortunately, the only cost-effective formulation suitable for tube administration (Glucophage powder, Merck) has been withdrawn in the UK, so in *practice* metformin is difficult to continue in enterally fed patients; if it has to be withdrawn for these practical reasons, patients will very likely need insulin: be vigilant.

---

*The Hands-on Guide to Diabetes Care in Hospital,* First Edition by David Levy.
© 2016 John Wiley & Sons, Ltd. Published 2016 by John Wiley & Sons, Ltd.

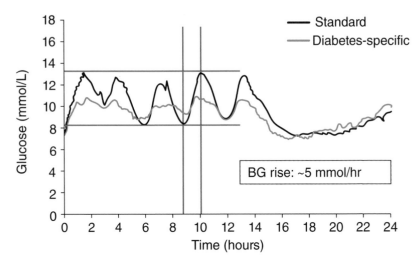

**Figure 28.1** Blood glucose levels after five enteral feeds given at 3-hourly intervals. Peak glucose values are about 2 mmol/L lower with diabetes-specific feeds, but there is no difference during non-feeding times, and any differences in achieved HbA$_{1c}$ would not be clinically meaningful. Blood glucose levels rise rapidly after starting standard feeds (~5 mmol/L in an hour). *Source*: Ceriello *et al.* 2009.

### Insulin treatment (Box 28.1)

Wherever possible start with and continue subcutaneous insulin in patients beginning enteral feeding. Even if a patient requires i.v. fluids, do not add the burden of VRIII.

### Subcutaneous insulin

*Note for US readers*: subcutaneous 'sliding scale' insulin (intermittent administration of variable doses of soluble insulin) is still widely used in the USA in acutely ill, general medical and surgical patients. However, there is current concern that it is less effective than traditional insulin regimens used out of hospital. Simple once-daily long-acting analogue insulin (glargine, Lantus, Sanofi-Aventis) is more effective than 6-hour sliding scale soluble insulin.

---

**Box 28.1**    Insulin treatment of enterally fed patients with diabetes

1. **Patients previously taking subcutaneous insulin at home:**
   a. **Continuous enteral feeding.** Give previous total daily dose as a single dose of long-acting analogue insulin, for example, Lantus at the start of the feed. Monitor blood glucose levels from 16–24 hours for evidence of waning of glycaemic effect; if this occurs, divide the dose into 2 equal 12-hourly injections. Alternatively, use 12-hourly isophane (NPH) insulin (e.g. Humulin I, Insuman Basal)
   b. **Intermittent enteral feeding.** Divide total dose by number of separate feeds. Give a high-mix biphasic insulin (e.g. Humalog Mix 50, Insuman Comb 50), 15–30 minutes before starting the feed; alternatively use modified basal-bolus regimen (see example below)
2. **Patients transferring from VRIII.** Give ~70% of the total previous 24-hour insulin requirement, either as basal, biphasic or modified basal-bolus insulin

3. **Patients naive to insulin, or previously on mixed insulin-non-insulin regimens.** Calculate starting dose as 0.5 U/kg body weight, and divide according to feeding regimen
4. **Discontinue non-insulin agents**, including sulphonylureas, which are likely to combine unpredictably with insulin to cause hypoglycaemia, but consider maintaining metformin, or adding it in, if there are no contraindications
5. **Review blood glucose and prescription charts daily.** Increase doses by 10% per day if necessary, in order to achieve capillary glucose measurements between 7 and 10 mmol/L, without hypoglycaemia
6. **Liaise closely with the inpatient diabetes team and the nutrition team**

**Example of a widely used feeding regimen:** a single feed lasting 12–16 hours, supplemented in the remaining hours (usually overnight) with water. In Type 2 patients, use a biphasic insulin preparation containing a high proportion (50%) of fast-acting to intermediate-acting insulin (e.g. Humalog Mix50, Insuman Comb 50). Give at 8-hourly intervals in equal doses, again at a total daily starting dose of approximately 0.5 U/ kg body weight. If BG levels still rise very rapidly, give the first dose 30 minutes before starting the feed. Ensure that the second dose is given strictly 8 hours after the first, so that when the feed is replaced with water there is a lower risk of hypoglycaemia. In Type 1 patients, who must not have an insulin-free period, use the same total dose: give half as long-acting basal insulin (Lantus, Levemir, Tresiba), and divide the remaining half into two doses of fast-acting analogue or soluble insulin given at 6–8 hourly intervals during the feed.

### Reference

Ceriello A, Lansink M, Rouws CH, van Laere KM, Frost GS. Administration of a new diabetes-specific enteral formula results in an improved 24h glucose profile in type 2 diabetic patients. *Diabetes Res Clin Pract.* 2009;84:259-66. PMID: 19307037.

### Further reading

Joint British Diabetes Societies for Inpatient Care. Glycaemic management during the inpatient enteral feeding of stroke patients with diabetes (June 2012). Available from: http://www.diabetologists-abcd.org.uk/JBDS/JBDS.htm (accessed on 24 August 2015).

# 29 Steroid-induced diabetes

**Top tip**

Test post-prandial CBG at least daily in all patients you start on systemic steroids.

**Key points**

- Steroid-induced diabetes is extremely common, and cannot be predicted by the usual risk factors for diabetes
- Steroids predominantly increase post-prandial, rather than fasting, glucose levels
- Hyperglycaemia starts within hours of an oral dose and is often severe. HHS is a real risk
- Only drugs with prompt post-prandial effects are of value (sulphonylureas, insulin, possibly GLP-1 analogues and DPP4 inhibitors)
- Most patients will need insulin, up to about 0.8 U/kg/day
- Remission from steroid-induced diabetes is unpredictable, so patients need follow-up after discharge

Steroid-induced diabetes is common, often severe, and usually requires insulin treatment. Steroids cause severe insulin resistance, mostly hepatic. Characteristically patients develop post-prandial hyperglycaemia immediately after starting steroid treatment, with only mild fasting hyperglycaemia, so prompt diagnosis requires daytime CBG monitoring; fasting BG levels are often completely normal. Because people of all phenotypes can develop diabetes after steroids, monitor CBG in everyone, even thin people.

Although the risks of diabetes are high with usual pharmacological doses of steroids, any doses higher than physiological may be associated with hyperglycaemia (**Table 29.1**). For some reason many doctors do not regard hydrocortisone as carrying the same risk of side effects as other steroids, but it is often given in high doses, so no steroid is without risk. Intra-articular steroids are very potent and often cause hyperglycaemia, but not inhaled steroids in adults, even in high doses.

**Table 29.1** Potencies of glucocorticoids and approximate physiological doses above which hyperglycaemia is a significant risk (see *British National Formulary*, section 6.3.2)

| Glucocorticoid | Approximate potency relative to hydrocortisone | Daily physiological dose (mg) |
|---|---|---|
| Hydrocortisone | 1 | 30 |
| Prednisolone | 4 | 7.5 |

*(Continued)*

*The Hands-on Guide to Diabetes Care in Hospital,* First Edition by David Levy.
© 2016 John Wiley & Sons, Ltd. Published 2016 by John Wiley & Sons, Ltd.

Table 29.1 *(Continued)*

| Glucocorticoid | Approximate potency relative to hydrocortisone | Daily physiological dose (mg) |
|---|---|---|
| Dexamethasone | 25 | 1.0 |
| Triamcinolone | 5 | 6 |
| Methylprednisolone | 5 | 6 |

## MANAGEMENT

### Patients with known diabetes

Although many diabetes medications will not be of much value in the severe hyperglycaemia caused by steroids, maintain all current medication, including metformin. However, it is only worthwhile increasing the doses of sulphonylureas and insulin.

### Diabetes treated with non-insulin agents (Chapter 24)

- Sulphonyulrea: start with gliclazide 80 mg twice daily, glimepiride 2 mg mane or glibenclamide 5 mg twice daily; if already taking a sulphonylurea, increase to maximum recommended doses: gliclazide 240 mg daily, glimepiride 4 mg daily, glibenclamide 15 mg daily
- Other glycaemic agents can be continued (including DPP4 inhibitors and GLP-1 analogues), but do not increase the doses
- Plan for early insulin treatment, certainly when CBG consistently >15 mmol/L, at which symptoms are likely:
  - Start with biphasic insulin 15–20 minutes before meals, e.g.
  - Humulin M3, NovoMix 30, Humalog Mix25 at 0.5 U/kg/day, divided approximately 2/3 before breakfast, 1/3 before evening meal
  - Alternatively three times daily biphasic insulin (Humalog Mix50, Insuman Comb 50) before meals if the patient is eating lunch (remember steroids will probably stimulate appetite)

Add in basal insulin at bedtime if fasting CBG >10. Start with the same number of units as the fasting glucose in mmol/L, and increase by 10% every day. There is a risk of fasting hypoglycaemia. On limited evidence, about 1/3 of the total daily dose of insulin will be basal/overnight, 2/3 prandial insulin to get good control.

### Insulin-treated diabetes

- Anticipate increased insulin requirements and **immediately increase each insulin dose by 25% when steroid treatment starts.** Because steroids increase insulin resistance, insulin-induced hypoglycaemia is unlikely
- Monitor post-prandial CBG levels every day and increase doses accordingly
- Involve the diabetes team as soon as possible

### Newly diagnosed steroid-induced diabetes

**Diagnosis:** random glucose >11 mmol/L (check HbA$_{1c}$ for evidence of undiagnosed diabetes, ≥6.5%, 48 mmol/mol)

Give a brief trial (2–3 days) of sulphonylurea (as above); increase the dose daily. If no effect, discontinue sulphonylurea and start insulin (as above).

### Further reading

Joint British Diabetes Societies for Inpatient Care Guideline. Management of hyperglycaemia and steroid (glucocorticoid) therapy (October 2014). Available from: www.diabetologists-abcd.org.uk/ JBDS/JBDS_IP_Steroids.pdf (accessed on 25 August 2015).

## 30 Safe discharge of patients from hospital

**Top tip**

Neither you nor the patient wants an unnecessary readmission with the same diabetes-related problem that caused their original admission. Discharge the patient carefully.

## DISCHARGE SUMMARY

A blow-by-blow account of your struggles with the patient's pH and serum magnesium levels is gratuitous, and irrelevant to primary care teams.

### Minimalist example

A 27 year old Type 1 patient admitted with vomiting after too much alcohol and omitting overnight Lantus insulin. Moderately severe DKA (pH 7.1) corrected within 24 hours.

Admission $HbA_{1c}$ was 9.3% (78 mmol/mol) – poor control. Seen by the inpatient diabetes team: educated about sick day rules and alcohol in diabetes, and written information given. Discharged on his usual insulin. Follow-up appointment arranged on Tuesday 7th December at 10-00 am in the diabetes centre.

### SICK DAY RULES

You should know these and their importance – Type 1 and insulin-treated Type 2 patients must never interrupt or discontinue insulin treatment (**Box 30.1**). Failure to observe the sick day rules is a frequent cause of DKA (**Chapter 9**).

---

**Box 30.1** Sick-day rules for people with insulin-treated diabetes

Infections, vomiting and diarrhoea are likely to raise your blood sugar levels. Even if you are not able to eat, you still need insulin, fluids and carbohydrate.

**Continue to take your usual insulin doses.**

Go to A&E straight away if:

- You vomit more than once or
- Have continuing diarrhoea or
- If your meter blood glucose readings show 'HI' (which usually means blood glucose greater than about 30 mmol/L).

---

*(Continued)*

---

*The Hands-on Guide to Diabetes Care in Hospital,* First Edition by David Levy.
© 2016 John Wiley & Sons, Ltd. Published 2016 by John Wiley & Sons, Ltd.

**Ketone measurements: go to A&E if:**
- You measure urine ketones and they are +++ or ++++
- You measure blood ketones and they are more than 3 mmol/L

If ketones are lower than this, continue to measure ketones every 4–6 hours, and treat as in the table below. If they increase to +++/++++ or blood ketones more than 3 mmol/L, go to A&E

| If you can eat | If you can't eat |
| --- | --- |
| **Food or carbohydrate** | |
| Usual meals | Take liquid carbohydrate every hour. Examples: ½ cup fruit juice (or half a small carton), ½ cup non-diet soft drink, ½ cup sports drink (e.g. Lucozade) |
| **Insulin** | |
| If blood glucose is 11—17, increase each insulin dose by 2 units | Take additional insulin: for example, 4 units of fast-acting or mixed insulin every 4 hours |
| If blood glucose is 17–22, increase each insulin dose by 4 units | |
| If blood glucose is more than 22, increase each insulin dose by 6 units | |
| **Fluids** | |
| Drink at least a cup of water or calorie-free fluid every hour (plain tea, caffeine-free soft drink, low-calorie fruit squash) | |
| **Glucose and ketone testing** | |
| Test blood glucose every 4–6 hours | Test blood glucose (and urine or blood ketones if possible) every 4 hours |

*Source*: Adapted from American Diabetes Association and Leicestershire Diabetes/DAFNE.

## MEDICATION

**People with established diabetes:**   'Is there anything you need to help you take your medication or insulin correctly as soon as you get home'?

**Newly diagnosed diabetes:**   Ensure the inpatient diabetes team has seen the patient in the last day or two to take into account any recent medication or insulin changes that may need reinforcing.

Ensure that insulin doses are meticulously noted in the discharge summary. Even if the patient is self-dosing, GPs and district nursing teams need to know the discharge insulin regimen and dosing in detail; district nurses will understandably not give insulin to patients unless the dose is specified. If district nurses or pharmacists need to contact you, then you have probably not written a clear prescription. Learn.

**Insulin delivery devices:**   If the patient is not self-administering insulin in hospital, the insulin delivery device – pen – isn't of importance, but it is very important when they are back home. Ward pharmacists will normally ensure that the correct device is dispensed, but check they haven't forgotten.

## FOLLOW-UP

Patients with acute diabetes problems will have outpatient follow-up with the diabetes nursing team – but always confirm this in the discharge summary and that the patient knows the appointment day, time and place. Routine medical outpatient appointments do not happen soon enough to be of value to the patient, unless there are long-term problems that also need tackling, for example, nephropathy, or a new medical problem. If there is a newly recognised problem, for example, ischaemic heart disease or proteinuria, arrange an appointment in the appropriate specialist clinic.

**Patients admitted with acute diabetic foot problems:**   Again, ensure that there is a firm arrangement for follow-up – which will vary according to your local circumstances, though most hospitals will have specialist podiatrists. Patients with chronic foot problems may not be punctilious outpatient attenders, but help by giving them written details about appointments. Bear in mind the visual impairment in patients with retinopathy and other eye problems – a black marker pen is often helpful.

### General practitioner follow-up
Don't ask GPs to do unreasonable things, and certainly nothing that you couldn't manage yourself, for example, adjusting insulin doses. Recognise practical difficulties as well: for example it is often quite difficult for patients to get urgent appointments with their GPs.

*Comment*:   the unfulfilled promise/superficial reassurance on discharge ('don't worry, you will get an appointment/follow-up for …' that then never happens) is a major problem that upsets people and is a potential hazard. We know you are busy, but do everything you can to 'make it happen'; it will probably take only a few minutes. You and your patient will certainly feel and probably be better for it. Diabetes is a long-term condition, and making it happen will probably do more to improve cooperation and 'compliance' than anything, especially in people who don't currently engage with diabetes services.

### Guidelines and flowchart for patients
http://www.leicestershirediabetes.org.uk/uploads//documents/Type1%20Sick_day_rules_InsulinV3.pdf
  http://www.leicestershirediabetes.org.uk/uploads//documents/Type2%20Sick_day_rules_InsulinV3.pdf (accessed on 25 August 2015)

# PART 6
# Important odds and ends

# 31 Technology in diabetes

**Key points**

- There is little high-tech equipment in use in diabetes – but the technology that is available is ubiquitous in the developed world
- Understand the value and limitations of point of care (POC) tests for capillary blood glucose and ketones
- Insulin cartridge pens are used by nearly every diabetic patient in the UK. Recognise the different varieties (disposable and reusable)
- Continuous subcutaneous insulin infusion (CSII) devices (insulin pumps) are widely used in Type 1 diabetes. They are valuable in inpatient care (emergency and elective)
- Know in outline the current status of pancreas, kidney-pancreas and islet-cell transplantation, and of the fully automated (closed-loop) insulin pump – patients are understandably interested in them, and you are likely to be asked
- Diabetes, particularly Type 1, has benefited over the past 30 years from continuous improvements in insulin delivery devices and portable capillary glucose (and ketone) measurements. Taken together, these rather undramatic changes have probably been more important than the better-known changes in insulin products themselves for the well-being and general improvement in outcomes seen across the developed world in Type 1, and to a lesser extent Type 2 diabetes

## CAPILLARY BLOOD GLUCOSE METERS

These all use whole capillary blood obtained by finger prick (use the sides of the pulp of the fingers, not the tip). In order to standardise the measurements, and also to make them comparable to venous plasma glucose levels – the laboratory standard – all meters now 'correct' readings to a venous plasma equivalent (around 11–12% higher). This is the reason for caution in interpreting measurements in severe anaemia (meter over-read) or polycythaemia (under).

### Hospital-based devices
Many hospitals now have networked systems and all BG measurements are centrally recorded and retrievable. The FreeStyle Precision Pro BG glucose range is 1.1–27.7 mmol/L (=500 mg/dL) and beta ketones <0.5–8.0 mmol/L.

### Devices for home blood glucose monitoring (HBGM)
There are dozens of devices, and they change or are updated continuously.

*The Hands-on Guide to Diabetes Care in Hospital,* First Edition by David Levy.
© 2016 John Wiley & Sons, Ltd. Published 2016 by John Wiley & Sons, Ltd.

### Accuracy in the hypoglycaemic range
Meters are designed to be extremely accurate in the hypoglycaemic range. Home meters read as low as 2.2 mmol/L, the hospital FreeStyle Precision Pro 1.1 mmol/L. They will not display a reading unless the blood sample has been applied correctly and in a sufficient amount. You do not need to repeat a meter reading for confirmation in the hypoglycaemic range before taking action.

### Accuracy in the hyperglycaemic range
The FreeStyle Precision Pro reads up to 500 mg/dL (=27.7 mmol/L). Above this the display will show >27.7 mmol/L (**Figure 31.1**), but the > sign can easily be overlooked. This is one situation in which SI unit users should be aware of the conversion factor between mmol/L and mg/dL (approximately 18). If you see a reading of 27.7 or thereabouts in the hospital record or observation chart, check laboratory glucose. It goes without saying that the laboratory result could be anywhere between 27.8 and 110 (the highest glucose measurement I have encountered).

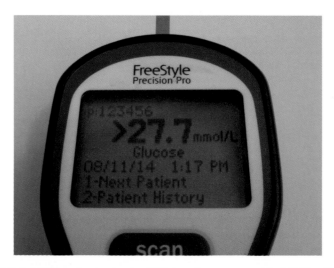

**Figure 31.1** Hospital-based meter showing CBG above its measurement limit (27.7 mol/L). The '>' sign is often omitted during transcription.

## URINALYSIS

Urinalysis, especially for ketones, is very important (significant ketonuria = insulin deficiency). Ensure it is done promptly in all patients with diabetes, preferably in the ED, and mandatorily if there is a suspicion of a hyperglycaemic emergency. Automated urinalysis is now universal in hospitals. Diagnosis is traditionally based on the 'plus system' (for example, significant ketonuria is defined as ≥2+); however modern urinalysis systems can be switched to a semi-quantitative output, and you may be given this, with no option to convert. The conversions (in the Siemens Clinitek system, widely used in the UK and USA) are shown in **Table 31.1**.

**Table 31.1** Comparison of semi-quantitative and 'plus' reporting scales for Clinitek urinalysis system

| Test | Units | Reported results | |
|------|-------|------------------|---|
| | | Semi-quantitative system | Plus system |
| **Glucose** | mmol/L | Negative | Negative |
| | | 5.5 | Trace |
| | | 14 | 1+ |
| | | 28 | 2+ |
| | | ≥55 | 3+ |
| **Ketone** | mmol/L | Negative | Negative |
| | | Trace | Trace |
| | | 1.5 | 1+ |
| | | 3.9 | 2+ |
| | | 7.8 | 3+ |
| | | ≥15.6 | 4+ |
| **Protein** | g/L | Negative | Negative |
| | | 0.15 | Low |
| | | 0.3 | 1+ |
| | | 1.0 | 2+ |
| | | 3.0 | 3+ |
| **Leucocytes** | Leu/µL | Negative | Negative |
| | | Ca 15 | Trace |
| | | Ca 70 | 1+ |
| | | Ca 125 | 2+ |
| | | Ca 500 | 3+ |
| **Nitrite** | | Negative | Negative |
| | | Positive | Positive |
| **Blood** | Ery/µL | Negative | Negative |
| | | Trace-lysed | Trace-lysed |
| | | Trace-intact | Trace-intact |
| | | Ca 25 | 1+ |
| | | Ca 80 | 2+ |
| | | Ca 200 | 3+ |

*Source*: Clinitek Operator's Manual (2004).

Urinary ketones detect acetone and acetoacetate, but not the most important ketone, β-OH butyrate (**Chapter 5**). However, this is relevant only in the resolution phase of DKA, when plasma β-OH butyrate may be low, having been oxidised to acetoacetate and acetone, while the latter two may increase in the urine.

## INSULIN DELIVERY DEVICES

Most insulin-using diabetic people in the UK use pen devices. Introduced in the early 1980s, they give reproducibly accurate dosing in single unit steps, and in some devices half-units. They all use 3-mL cartridges and can deliver up to 60 or 80 units as a single dose. Most UK patients use disposable pens for convenience, but refillable pens are robust and can last for many years.

As with blood glucose meters, designs change frequently. **Figure 31.2** shows examples of refillable insulin pens and **Figure 31.3** shows disposable pens.

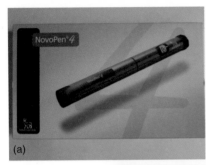

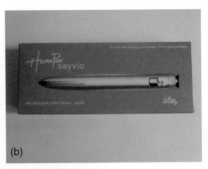

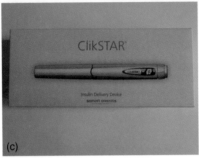

**Figure 31.2** Refillable insulin pens. (a) Novopen 4 (Novo Nordisk). (b) HumaPen Savvio (Lilly). (c) ClikSTAR (Sanofi-Aventis).

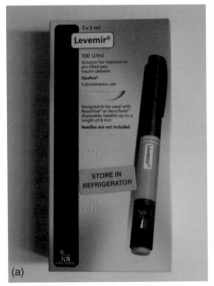

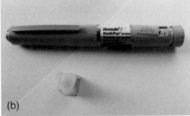

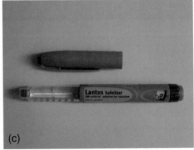

**Figure 31.3** Disposable insulin pens. (a) Flexpen (Novo Nordisk). (b) KwikPen (Lilly). (c) SoloSTAR (Sanofi-Aventis).

### Injection needles

An EU safety directive (implementation May 2014) aiming to reduce needle-stick injuries includes the requirement for specific guarded insulin injection needles in hospital. Patients giving their own insulin injections can use standard unguarded needles that they bring into hospital (though they are required to dispose of them in a sharps container supplied to them for their use alone). All insulin injections given by hospital staff will require the newly designed disposable pen needles (BD AutoShield Duo, 5-mm length; **Chapter 33, Figure 31.3**).

## INSULIN PUMPS (Continuous Subcutaneous Insulin Infusion, CSII; Chapter 21)

Widely, in some countries almost universally, used in Type 1 diabetes, insulin pumps are increasing in the UK. They aim to improve glycaemic control by more closely mimicking physiological insulin secretion with a single rapid-acting analogue insulin given in two ways:

- Basal insulin delivered continuously at a low rate, usually around 1 U/hr
- Bolus insulin delivered pre-meal in doses calculated using the principles of carbohydrate counting

They are now highly sophisticated devices which can be precisely programmed to deliver variable basal insulin rates. Patients often report improved well-being, and there are strong indications of modest overall improvement in glycaemic control, compared with basal-bolus insulin. Patients with frequent hypoglycaemic episodes and recurrent admissions with DKA are often helped.

Current insulin pumps can't deliver insulin automatically – a widespread misconception. They require as much self-care as patients using MDI, and starting pump treatment needs a formal education program. While not yet approved for Type 2 diabetes, limited trial evidence is encouraging.

A new generation of disposable 'patch' pumps dispenses with the need for insulin lines and complex set-up procedures, and these are likely to be increasingly used (**Figure 31.4**).

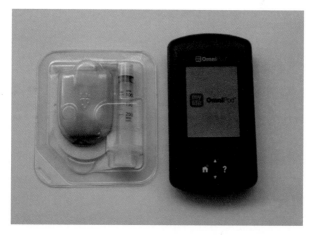

**Figure 31.4** A 'patch' pump (OmniPod Insulin Management System, Ypsomed). On the left is the single-use pump, usually applied to the abdomen, and which is discarded and a new one applied once the single-fill insulin reservoir containing 200 units is finished (about 2–4 days). Right: the separate remote control device for the pump with an integrated blood glucose meter.

## Inpatient management of patients with insulin pumps

Patients using insulin pumps are usually highly motivated and well trained in their use. They will almost certainly know more than you about their treatment; trust them. There are no agreed guidelines for their use in hospital, but bear the following in mind:

- Contact the diabetes team as soon as possible (some hospitals have 24 hour specialist nurse contacts)
- Critically ill patients with non-diabetes-related illnesses should be transferred to VRIII, and pump treatment discontinued
- Patients with DKA should continue basal insulin alone (no boluses) until they are eating
- Patients for elective surgery can also continue basal insulin; careful liaison with anaesthetists and the diabetes team is a must
- Insulin pumps are affected by X-rays. A pump can be discontinued for up to an hour for a relatively short procedure; if longer than that, use VRIII

## EXISTING AND FUTURE TECHNOLOGY WHICH YOU MAY BE ASKED ABOUT

### (Whole) pancreas transplantation for Type 1 diabetes

'Am I eligible'?

'No', unless:

- they have Type 1 diabetes and are relatively young (e.g. <60 years)
- there is advanced CKD or ESRD (and therefore eligible for simultaneous pancreas and kidney transplantation) and there is also unstable diabetes (e.g. hypoglycaemia unawareness or frequent DKA – or both ('brittle' diabetes) resulting in frequent hospitalisation)
- there are other associated recurrent problems, for example, advanced gastroparesis

The long-term discipline needed for permanent immunosuppression, frequent specialist hospital visits and the potential complications of immunosuppression (especially cancers) mean that only about 200 people a year in the United Kingdom come to any form of pancreas transplantation. About 80% are simultaneous pancreas and kidney transplant, 10–20% pancreas-after-kidney, and 5% pancreas alone. Operative outcomes are good for such a formidable transplant procedures (e.g. 85–90% 5-year patient survival) and pancreas graft survival is about 70% at 5 years in the best centres.

### Islet-cell transplantation

Although a much simpler procedure than whole-pancreas transplantation, islet-cell transplantation is less predictably successful (around 50% insulin-independence at 1 year), and the outstanding results obtained in Edmonton, Canada, have not been emulated in less experienced centres. Immunosuppression and meticulous long-term follow-up are needed. Fewer than 40 patients in the UK had islet transplantations by 2012. It should be regarded as a treatment still under intensive investigation.

### The artificial pancreas

Much-publicised. The ultimate aim is a closed-loop system, in which continuous (subcutaneous, interstitial) glucose monitoring results are fed to an insulin infusion pump (or more likely an insulin-glucagon dual pump) which will deliver subcutaneous hormones automatically using an advanced algorithm with minimal patient intervention. For most

Type 1 patients such a device holds out the greatest hope for a 'cure', because it is technology- and not transplant-based. The first report of a successful trial of such a device in adult and adolescent outpatients was published in 2014. Commercial development is likely to occupy another 5 years, but there has been remarkable progress in this field over a relatively short period.

## Continuous glucose monitoring devices

Although you are unlikely to encounter inpatients using these devices, they are in widespread use, both for diagnostic purposes and increasingly as sophisticated replacements for simple finger prick home blood glucose monitoring. They rely on interstitial fluid glucose monitoring using a dynamic glucose-oxidase sensor, implanted simply and almost painlessly in the subcutaneous tissue, usually the arm. Because glucose levels have to equilibrate with blood, interstitial glucose levels lag behind blood glucose by ~10–15 minutes. While this limitation will be significant in the development of the closed-loop feedback system, it is fine for routine clinical use.

Importantly, continuous monitoring of glucose has increased our knowledge of minute-to-minute variation in glucose levels and the factors that affect them. Illustrations can act as a timely corrective to our imaginations, especially the flatline fallacy.

### Blinded glucose monitors (e.g. iPro2; Medtronic)

Data are not shown to patients, and can only be visualised on downloading. Sensors function for up to 7 days. Examples are shown in **Figure 31.5**.

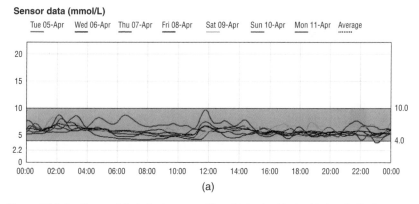

**Figure 31.5** Continuous (blinded) glucose profiles obtained with the Medtronic iPro2 system. X-axis, clock time, midnight-to-midnight; Y-axis, glucose readings (shaded range 4–10 mmol/L), operating range 2–20 mmol/L. A non-diabetic profile is shown in (a): glucose levels after meals can reach nearly 10 mmol/L, but most values are consistently between 4 and 7 mmol/L. (b) well-controlled Type 1 diabetes, with reasonably stable values during the day. Note the two nights with prolonged hypoglycaemia (values around 3 mmol/L). (c) poorly controlled Type 1 diabetes, with large post-prandial excursions after breakfast and evening meal, and frequent hypoglycaemic episodes (BG <4).

*(Continued)*

**Sensor data (mmol/L)**

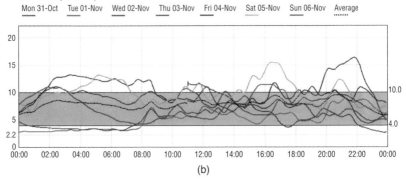

(b)

**Sensor data (mmol/L)**

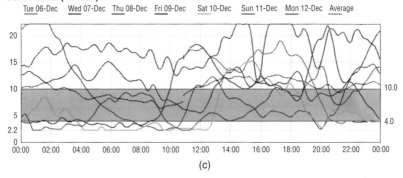

(c)

**Figure 31.5** *(Continued)*

## Ambulatory glucose profile (e.g. Abbot FreeStyle Libre) (Figure 31.6)

Data are always available to patients. The detector doubles as a conventional glucose meter. There is access to a graphical display of dynamic glucose changes. Arrows on the display indicate the trend of glucose levels, but there are currently no audible alarms. Sensors function for 14 days. They will be widely used in routine clinical practice by patients, especially Type 1 patients.

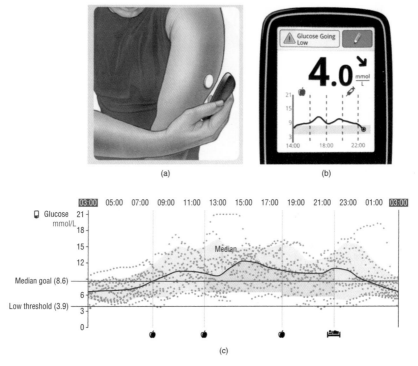

(a)

(b)

(c)

**Figure 31.6** Abbott FreeStyle Libre ambulatory glucose meter. (a) The sensor, which lasts for 14 days is inserted subcutaneously in the upper arm. The detector displays an instantaneous glucose reading once it is placed near the sensor. (b) The detector displays the glucose value and its trend and plots a graph of values. (c) One of the sophisticated download outputs, in a female Type 1 patient (duration 8 years) using a pump. The shaded area represents the 10th and 90th percentile limits of readings over the 14-day duration of a sensor. $HbA_{1c}$ at the time was 6.9% (52 mmol/L), with almost no hypoglycaemia, so this represents optimum control obtainable with current technology and self-care. From the point of view of the hospital practitioner, recognise that the upper 90th percentile limit during the day, even in this remarkably well-controlled individual exceeds 15 mmol/L after meals, but she will almost certainly not develop significant microvascular complications over her lifetime. Even if control deteriorates (e.g. to an $HbA_{1c}$ of 8% (64 mmol/mol) the legacy effect of the period of good control will significantly reduce her risk of micro- and macrovascular complications, and death from diabetes-related causes.

# 32 Inpatient screening schedule

**Key points**

- Take the opportunity of an acute admission with diabetes to screen sensibly for meaningful diabetic complications (taking into account age, duration of diabetes and comorbidities)
- Urinalysis for proteinuria, and a foot examination are mandatory

Screen patients for complications, especially patients with known diabetes admitted as an emergency – they are likely not to be attending their practice-based clinics and are at higher risk. Primary care annual reviews involve:

- Routine biochemistry, fasting lipids and urine for ACR
- Foot examination
- Education
- Photographic retinal screening usually at a local centre, usually reported by trained screeners. Neither reports nor the photographs themselves are currently accessible through hospital systems. Patients may not accurately remember their last appointment. Patients under care of hospital eye clinics will have advanced retinopathy, other eye pathology or both – advanced retinopathy is a reasonably reliable marker of other vascular complications, especially nephropathy and neuropathy

Most patients living locally will have some laboratory results available. $HbA_{1c}$ measurements tend, depressingly, to track reliably with time, in other words do not hugely change (unless the results are at the time of diagnosis; $HbA_{1c}$ in Type 2 diabetes tends to normalise for 6–12 months after diagnosis, then gradually climb). Most Type 1 patients and many Type 2 patients using insulin and/or with advanced complications will be known to the diabetes team, especially the diabetes specialist nurses (**Chapter 6**). Contact them: they will often be able to give you a useful summary of not only the patient's medical condition, but also their social and family circumstances.

Use the guidance below flexibly and with sensitivity, especially in patients with cancer and dementia. On the other hand there are especially vulnerable groups of patients (**Table 32.1**):

**Table 32.1** Groups of people with diabetes at risk of new or additional complications, or whose care can be compromised by their socio-economic status and deprivation

| Type 1 diabetes | Type 2 diabetes |
| --- | --- |
| • Admitted with DKA, especially recurrent<br>• Admitted with hypoglycaemia, especially recurrent | Admitted with HHS<br>Admitted with ACS |

*(Continued)*

*The Hands-on Guide to Diabetes Care in Hospital,* First Edition by David Levy.
© 2016 John Wiley & Sons, Ltd. Published 2016 by John Wiley & Sons, Ltd.

**Table 32.1** (*Continued*)

| Type 1 diabetes | Type 2 diabetes |
|---|---|
| Gastroparesis | Patients taking long-term antipsychotic medication |
| Eating disorder, especially anorexia<br>Homeless, itinerant, drug users, alcoholics<br>Severe psychiatric illness<br>Duration >10 years, especially if poorly controlled (risk of microvascular complications)<br>Duration >20 years, especially if currently >50 years old (risk of macrovascular complications, especially coronary heart disease) | |
| Patients with stick-positive proteinuria (≥1+) | |
| Patients admitted with foot ulceration | |
| Patients in the hospital eye clinic | |
| Dialysis or low clearance clinic patients | |

## FOCUSED CLINICAL EXAMINATION (Figure 32.1)

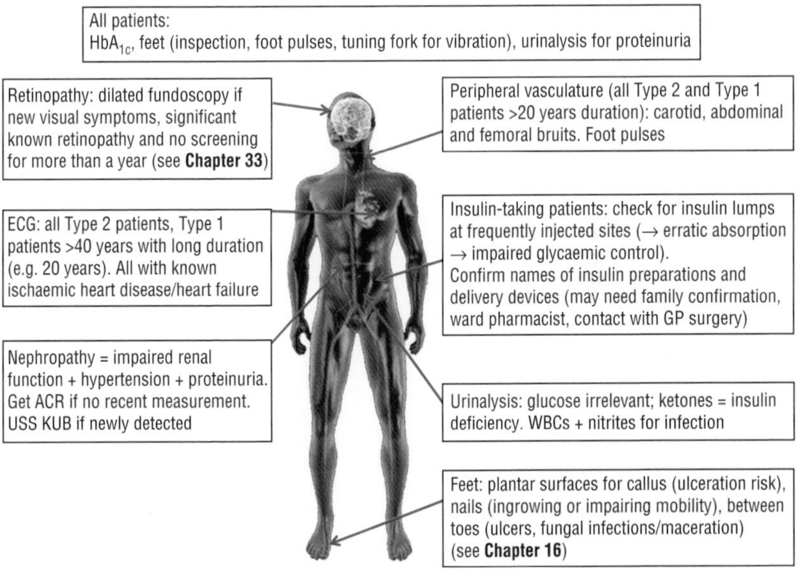

All patients:
$HbA_{1c}$, feet (inspection, foot pulses, tuning fork for vibration), urinalysis for proteinuria

Retinopathy: dilated fundoscopy if new visual symptoms, significant known retinopathy and no screening for more than a year (see **Chapter 33**)

Peripheral vasculature (all Type 2 and Type 1 patients >20 years duration): carotid, abdominal and femoral bruits. Foot pulses

ECG: all Type 2 patients, Type 1 patients >40 years with long duration (e.g. 20 years). All with known ischaemic heart disease/heart failure

Insulin-taking patients: check for insulin lumps at frequently injected sites (→ erratic absorption → impaired glycaemic control).
Confirm names of insulin preparations and delivery devices (may need family confirmation, ward pharmacist, contact with GP surgery)

Nephropathy = impaired renal function + hypertension + proteinuria. Get ACR if no recent measurement. USS KUB if newly detected

Urinalysis: glucose irrelevant; ketones = insulin deficiency. WBCs + nitrites for infection

Feet: plantar surfaces for callus (ulceration risk), nails (ingrowing or impairing mobility), between toes (ulcers, fungal infections/maceration) (see **Chapter 16**)

**Figure 32.1** Some features of the general examination of inpatients with diabetes.

# 33 Practical procedures

**Key skills**

- Capillary blood glucose testing using a hospital-based system
- Capillary blood glucose testing using a home meter
- Giving a subcutaneous insulin injection
- Practical wound dressing for a diabetic foot ulcer
- Direct ophthalmoscopy

The few practical procedures in diabetes are well worth knowing about. It is unlikely you will be regularly called on to do any of them, but you should be able to help give a subcutaneous insulin injection if a patient needs one and has their own insulin equipment. However, they will use standard insulin needles, and not the hospital safety devices. Don't re-sheathe the insulin needle with the narrow cap after giving an injection, but use the larger plastic cap to screw off the needle and dispose of it.

## CAPILLARY BLOOD GLUCOSE TESTING USING A HOSPITAL-BASED SYSTEM (Figure 33.1)

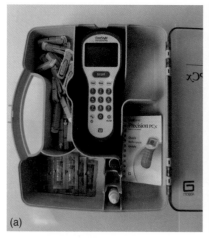
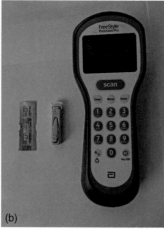

(a)      (b)

**Figure 33.1** Testing capillary blood glucose using a hospital-based system (FreeStyle Precision Pro [Abbott]). For purposes of quality control, security and traceability, the user needs a barcode, allocated after appropriate training, which is scanned before each test (e), followed by a scan of the individual blood strip (f). Get blood from the side, not the tip, of a finger (i, j).

*The Hands-on Guide to Diabetes Care in Hospital,* First Edition by David Levy.
© 2016 John Wiley & Sons, Ltd. Published 2016 by John Wiley & Sons, Ltd.

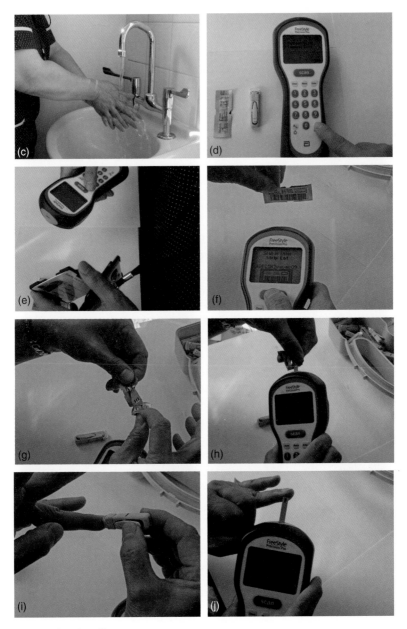

**Figure 33.1** *(Continued)*

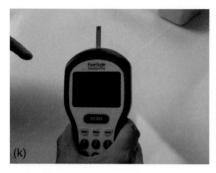
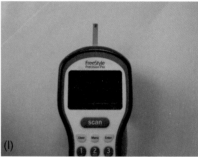

**Figure 33.1** *(Continued)*

## CAPILLARY BLOOD GLUCOSE TESTING USING A TYPICAL HOME DEVICE (Figure 33.2)

Many patients will bring their own blood glucose testing devices – of which there are countless varieties – into hospital. If you are concerned about mild hypoglycaemia, for example, it may be quicker to ask the patient to test their own blood glucose level in front of you. BG testing is very simple and you should be able to do it reliably yourself if circumstances require it.

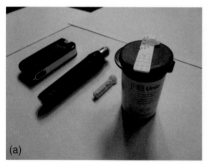
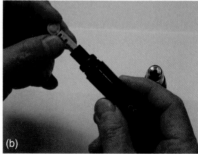

**Figure 33.2** CBG testing with a meter designed for home use (Unio, Ypsomed), (a) L to R: Meter, finger pricker, lancet, tub of testing sticks. There are dozens of devices for finger pricking. Hospitals have single-use items (see **Figure 33.1 (i)**). (b), (c) Assemble finger pricker and lancet. (d), (e) Inserting the test strip (side-loading in this case) starts the meter. (f), (g) Small blood drop obtained from the side of the finger pulp to reduce discomfort. (h), (i) All meters now start testing automatically as soon as sufficient blood has been taken up by capillary action. (j) Most meters display the result after 5 seconds.

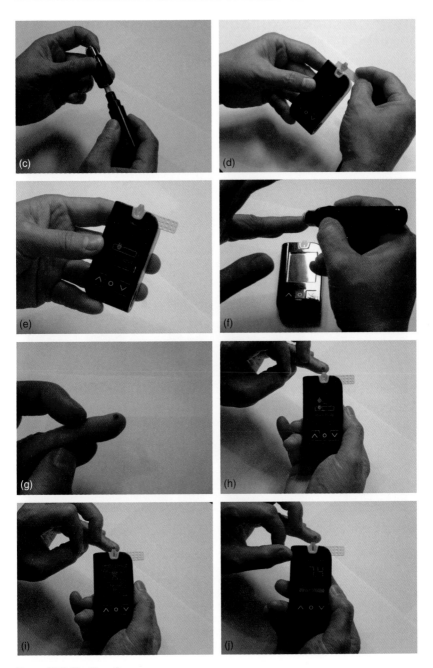

**Figure 33.2** (*Continued*)

# GIVING A SUBCUTANEOUS INSULIN INJECTION (Figure 33.3)

The general principles apply to all subcutaneous injections. Skin cleaning before giving insulin injections is no longer recommended.

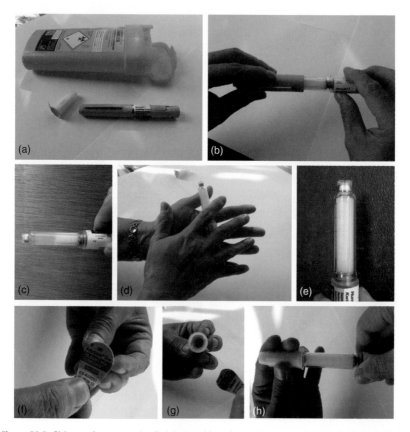

**Figure 33.3** Giving a subcutaneous insulin injection. (a) Insulin pen (here containing cloudy isophane (NPH) insulin [Humulin I]), BD AutoShield Duo with integral 5-mm needle, sharps disposal box. (b), (c), The heavy crystals of insulin result in separation from the diluent. These insulins are usual given every 24 hours, and they need resuspension every day. They are the only cloudy insulins in regular use: all others are clear and do not need resuspension. (d), (e), Roll the insulin pen between the hands (don't shake) about 12–15 times until the suspension is uniformly milky. (f), (g), (h), (i) Remove the paper tab from the insulin needle, screw the assemblage to the insulin pen and remove the outer plastic cap. (j), (k) Do an 'air shot' to make sure any dead space in the pen and needle has been removed: dial 2 units, and inject to zero. (l) Dial up the intended dose, in this case 15 units (numbering on the visible window is usually in even numbers only). (m), (n) Press lightly against the skin and perpendicularly to the skin surface. Injections are best given in the abdomen, avoiding the immediate periumbilical area, any skin lesions, bruises from previous injections, and insulin 'lumps' from repeated areas of previous injections — all of which are likely to cause erratic absorption of insulin. Inject to zero, and hold the pen in the skin for a few seconds before withdrawing it. (o), (p) Unscrew the needle and dispose. (q) Recap the insulin pen (clicks on).

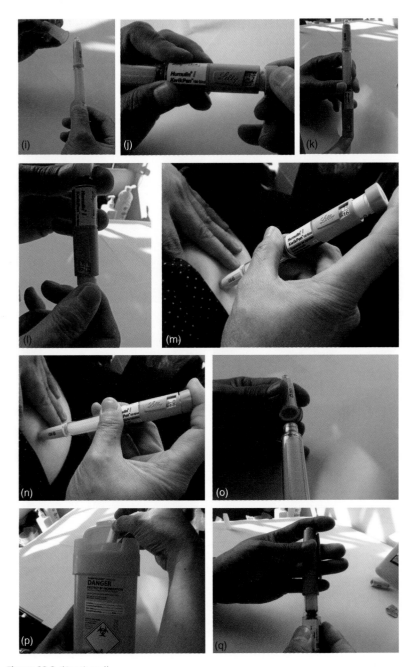

**Figure 33.3** *(Continued)*

## PRACTICAL WOUND DRESSING FOR A DIABETIC FOOT ULCER (Figure 33.4)

Nursing staff may ask you to prescribe appropriate dressings, usually in the acute situation before the multidisciplinary diabetes team or tissue viability team have been able to review the patient. If you take a dressing down to examine a foot lesion you should be able to either replace it yourself with a simple one, or advise colleagues if they need help.

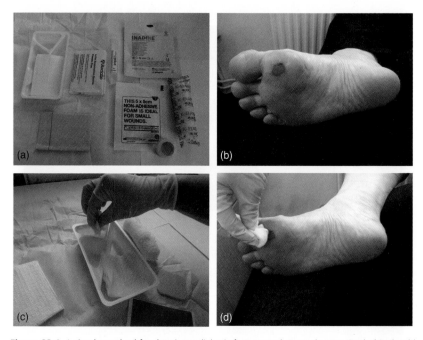

**Figure 33.4** A simple method for dressing a diabetic foot wound. Properly organised, this should take less than about 10 minutes. (a) Use a standard dressing pack and aseptic technique. In addition (right) – iodine dressing (e.g. Inadine), nonadhesive foam dressing (e.g. Allevyn), adhesive tape and K Band bandage. (There will be many local differences in brands etc.). (b) Typical position of a neuropathic ulcer to be dressed. (c), (d) Use saline-soaked dressing to thoroughly clean the wound. More specialist cleaning and debridement can be performed after detailed assessment (especially sharp debridement with a scalpel if there is adherent exudate). It is conventional to take a swab for microbiology from the deepest part of the ulcer, but the results are of no clinical value (**Chapter 16**). (e), (f) Cut the iodine dressing to a size just sufficient to cover the wound. If the patient is sensitive to iodine, use a simple nonadhesive dry dressing. (g) Cover with a nonadhesive foam dressing cut to size if necessary. (h), (i) Cover lightly but firmly with the conforming bandage. Its role is not protective (in this acute stage patients must be on bedrest) but simply to hold the other dressings in place, so do not go to inordinate lengths, even if they are provided (for the cost-conscious: current BNF price 19p). (j) Use minimal adhesive tape and do not attach it to skin, as it can cause damage in the neuropathic foot. (k) Completed dressing.

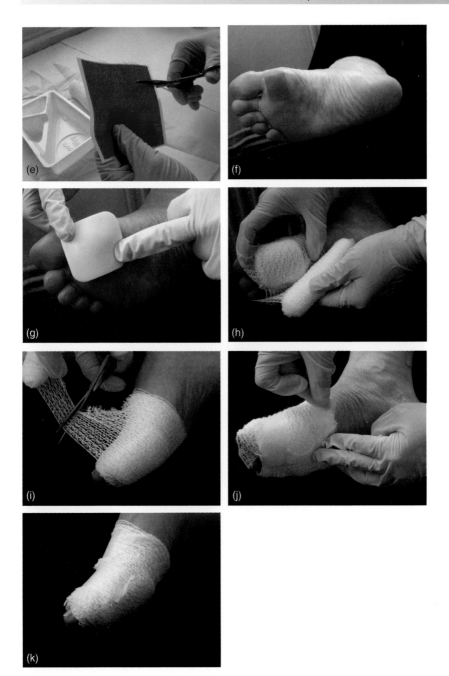

**Figure 33.4** *(Continued)*

## DIRECT OPHTHALMOSCOPY (Figure 33.5)

A key skill, critically important and not just in diabetes. You cannot diagnose raised intracranial pressure or properly examine a patient with accelerated hypertension without fundoscopy. Patients with diabetes are generally helpful subjects, as they frequently have eye examinations; even those who attend just for annual nonmydriatic eye screening will be well used to bright lights and fixing their gaze. Patients under the hospital eye service will have experienced dilating drops on many occasions.

Ophthalmoscopy is a simple procedure but in practice often frustrating. Tropicamide eye drops are sometimes not available when and where you need them, and finding a fully charged ophthalmoscope isn't always easy, either. Be patient.

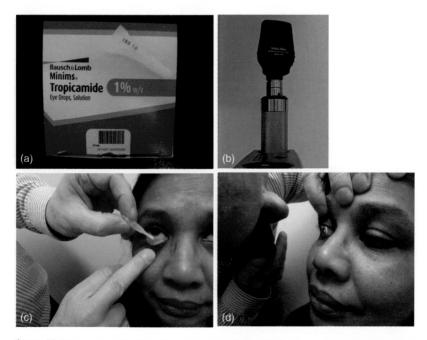

**Figure 33.5** (a) Tropicamide 1% drops in individual dispensers. They sting: warn the patient. (b) Wherever possible use a full-size, fully-charged ophthalmoscope. (c) Instil a single drop into the lower conjunctival sac of each eye, warning the patient that it will sting for a short time. Don't apply directly to the cornea. It will take up to 20 minutes for full pupillary dilatation. (d) Adjust the ophthalmoscope, if necessary, for your refraction.

Keys to getting a good view of the fundus are the following:

- Try to examine the patient at the same level as you (for example, if possible, ask them to sit with their legs over the edge of a bed and raise it)
- Hold the ophthalmoscope horizontally so that you can get close to the patient's eye
- Gently elevate the upper eyelid, especially in older people who may have some ptosis

- Use minimum light intensity at all times to reduce discomfort for the patient; start at low intensity and gradually increase it as necessary
- Ensure the patient looks straight ahead and doesn't follow the light
- Don't tire the patient or yourself
- In examining for diabetic retinopathy the peripheral fundus is more important than the disc, but locate the disc first and move outwards along the main blood vessels, where early retinopathy tends to cluster. Patients often have a few thin blood vessels running across the margins of the disc; disc new vessels *never* occur by themselves – there will always be obvious retinopathy elsewhere (new vessels are difficult to detect on direct ophthalmoscopy in any case). Most inpatients are Type 2, so try to locate the macula (2 disc diameters lateral to the lateral margin of the optic disc); any exudates or haemorrhages in this area (which is avascular) may impair vision – get an urgent eye review for ocular coherence tomography (OCT), which is the only reliable way to detect macular oedema.

# 34 On-call guide to hyperglycaemic emergencies

## HYPEROSMOLAR HYPERGLYCAEMIC STATE (HHS) – NO LONGER CALLED HONK

### Key points

- HHS is different from DKA: make the diagnosis
- **Causes**: new-onset T2DM, worsening known T2DM (often insidious), steroid-induced or exacerbated, not taking diabetes medication (often for several weeks)
- ↑Osmolarity →↑obtundation and ↑blood viscosity, ↑↑risk of VTE and arterial thrombosis: full anticoagulation if osmolarity >140 and no contraindications
- Use gentler fluid and insulin than in DKA: risk of osmotic demyelination if rapid [Na⁺] shifts
- Manage on Emergency Admissions Unit: ICU opinion if bad biochemistry or organ failure: ask diabetes team to review early

### Biochemical features

- Hyperosmolarity (calculate: $2[Na^+] + [urea] + [glucose]$); present if >320, severe if >340
- Worse hyperglycaemia than in DKA (BG usually >30, sometimes 50–100)
- Usually AKI (e.g. Cr >200)
- Allow trace urinary ketones or 1+. If heavier ketonuria, then DKA or mixed picture
- $HCO_3^-$, venous pH both normal.
- Hypernatraemia very common: admission [Na⁺] lab result is often low, but always correct for glucose at the time – **+1 mmol/L [Na⁺] for each 4 mmol/L glucose**

### Laboratory investigations

- Laboratory glucose (CAUTION: hospital meters read only up to about 27.8)
- U+Es every 6–8 hours (watch for rapid changes in corrected [Na⁺]: get advice if >155)
- Laboratory glucose until in range of hospital meters (<28)
- Infection screen and CRP (examine feet for ulcers)
- Sick/AKI: lactate, CK, amylase, troponin, ECG
- ECG and troponin
- $HbA_{1c}$

*The Hands-on Guide to Diabetes Care in Hospital*, First Edition by David Levy.
© 2016 John Wiley & Sons, Ltd. Published 2016 by John Wiley & Sons, Ltd.

## Fluids

- **0.9% NaCl**. If glucose-corrected [Na⁺] >150, alternate Hartmann's or PlasmaLyte and 0.45% NaCl (or 0.9% NaCl) after initial 1–2 L of 0.9% NaCl
- Fluid can precede starting insulin by 1–2 hours
- Suggested fluid regime: fluid challenge if hypotensive, then 1 L + KCl over 2 hours, 4 hours, 4 hours, 6 hours, 6 hours, 8 hours (~6 L over ~30 hours)

## Insulin

- LOW rate, for example, start at 2 U/hr (NOT 6 U/hr: aim to reduce BG gradually by about 3 mmol/hr (difficult). 2012 JBDS guideline: insulin not required unless CBG isn't falling, but don't do this yet, because there is a risk the insulin start will be delayed because of mis-communication etc.
- 6U/hr high-dose insulin regimen + 10% glucose (as used in DKA) isn't needed – no ketosis to suppress

## Continuing management

- Often sick, elderly, and require careful management: ensure first 24 hours is in Emergency Admissions Unit
- Recovery can be slow: use VRIII until eating
- No need for NBM unless another reason
- Most new T2DM are fine on gliclazide 40–80 mg bd (+ metformin 500 mg bd if no contraindications)
- Insulin if in doubt, or major weight loss pre-admission, BMI <25, poor control (e.g. A1C >9%, 75 mmol/mol) on maximum non-insulin agents
- Be clinically vigilant and repeat biochemistry frequently: HHS still carries a mortality

# DIABETIC KETOACIDOSIS (DKA)

### Key points

- DKA is a state of **insulin deficiency**: fluids to correct the severe dehydration, and insulin to suppress ketogenesis are more important than lowering BG
- **Diagnosis** requires all of:
  - **D**iabetes (BG ~20–30, but can be lower in starving, vomiting or pregnant patients)
  - **K**etosis: urinary ketones ≥2+ or capillary ketones (β-OH butyrate) >1.5 mmol/L (usually >4)
  - **A**cidosis: venous pH <7.3 ± $HCO_3^-$ ≤18 (pH: severe <7.0, moderate 7.0–7.24, mild 7.25–7.30)
- **Causes**: decompensated known T1DM (infection, GI upset, alcohol intoxication, recreational drugs, discontinuing insulin when not eating – i.e. not sticking to sick-day rules), new-onset T1DM (now unusual except in kids)
- 'Flatbush' diabetes characteristic of overweight middle-aged black males (actually T2DM, but presents with DKA and initially insulin requiring)
- **Manage on AAU**: ICU advice if ↓GCS, pH <7.0, shocked, adolescent, pregnant, elderly + comorbidities
- **Risks**: hypokalaemia, slow resolution of acidosis and ketosis, delayed discharge

### Lab investigations (see HHS)
Also:

- Venous blood gases
- Correct [Na⁺] for prevailing glucose (see HHS)
- If sick or very acidotic: amylase (allow up to 3 times ULN), CK, phosphate + Mg
- HbA$_{1c}$
- Infection screen (examine feet): WBC commonly ↑ as a result of DKA itself, but always look for infection; acidosis also causes abdominal pain, but ~20% have abdo pathology, especially pancreatitis; get abdominal CT

### Fluids

- 0.9% NaCl. Hartmann's or PlasmaLyte do not resolve DKA quicker than NaCl
- Suggested fluid regime fluid challenge if hypotensive, then NaCl 1 L over 1 hour, 2 hours, 2 hours, 4 hours, 4 hours, 6 hours (~6 L over ~20 hours)
- Low [K⁺] is a problem (acidosis and insulin): gases will give you approx. [K⁺], then 20–40 mmol/L KCl
- **Once CBG <14, ADD separate infusion of 10% glucose** at 100 mL/hr (no sooner than 2–3 hours)

### Insulin

- Prescribe any long-acting s.c. insulin at usual dose
- i.v. insulin at 6 U/hr (JBDS: suggests 0.1 U/kg/hr, but it is difficult to weigh patients in ED and may be too much in heavy patients)
- Maintain i.v. insulin at 6 U/hr to suppress ketosis once CBG <14 and 10% glucose has started
- Continue triple infusion until capillary ketones <0.5
- If drinking but not eating continue VRIII with 5% glucose; if not eating or drinking continue VRIII with separate NaCl + glucose (don't use 'flip-flop')

### Monitor

- CBG every hour
- VBG every 1–2 hours until pH normal
- Capillary ketones every 4–6 hours until <0.5
- U+Es every 6–8 hours

### Continuing management

- Patients can eat and drink when able (no need for nil by mouth)
- Only start s.c. insulin when biochem normal and capillary ketones <0.5 mmol/L; discontinue i.v. insulin 30 minutes after s.c. Do not discontinue i.v. insulin late in the day; aim to continue VRIII overnight and discontinue after breakfast next day
- Ensure diabetes team review as early as possible (preferably on admission)

# Index

*The Hands-on Guide to Diabetes Care in Hospital,* First Edition by David Levy.
© 2016 John Wiley & Sons, Ltd. Published 2016 by John Wiley & Sons, Ltd.